The Revolutionary 7-Unit Low Fat Diet

The Revolutionary 7-Unit Low Fat Diet

The Diet That Lets You Enjoy Pasta, Bread, Potatoes—and Even a Drink—While Losing Up to 7 Pounds in 7 Days

by

JEAN CARPER and **AUDREY EYTON**

Introduction by
HENRY A. JORDAN, M.D.

RAWSON, WADE PUBLISHERS, INC.
NEW YORK

Library of Congress Cataloging in Publication Data
Carper, Jean.
The revolutionary 7-unit low fat diet.
Includes index.
1. Low-fat diet. I. Eyton, Audrey. II. Title.
III. Title: 7-unit low fat diet.
RM237.7.C36   613.2'5   80-5982
ISBN 0-89256-156-4   AACR2

Published simultaneously in Canada by McClelland and Stewart, Ltd.
Composition by American–Stratford Graphic Services,
Brattleboro, Vermont
Manufactured by Fairfield Graphics, Fairfield, Pennsylvania

Designed by Jacques Chazaud

First Edition

Medical professionals and nutritionists generally agree that the reduction of fat in the diet is not only a sure-fire means of losing weight but is also vitally important to overall health. Yet we point out that this or any other diet should be followed only under a doctor's supervision.

CONTENTS

PART I

THE 7-UNIT LOW FAT DIET

A New Approach to Weight Loss

Before
You Begin This Book

AN INTRODUCTION
BY DR. HENRY A. JORDAN

Dr. Jordan is a psychiatrist who has specialized for many years in the research and treatment of obesity and has become recognized as one of America's foremost medical experts on weight problems. As Clinical Associate Professor of Psychiatry he directs a research laboratory, investigating human eating habits at the University of Pennsylvania, where he conducts training programs for doctors, psychologists and nutritionists.

Dr. Jordan is the head of the Institute for Behavioral Education in King of Prussia, Pennsylvania. He is a member of the American Psychiatric Association, Eastern Psychological Association and the Philadelphia College of Physicians.

When I first saw the English edition of this diet, two years ago, I was amazed by the ingenious system that had been devised to tackle that major single cause of the great Western weight problem—our overconsumption of fats. Few modern medical experts would disagree that fats, more than any other foods, are the culprits behind our epidemic of obesity.

With this system, here, at last, was something new in weight reduction. Not "just another diet" based on some current fad, but a completely new approach which might realistically make a difference. An approach to which doctors and scientists, working in the field of obesity, could give their full support.

The latest reports on obesity in the U.S. are alarming. They indicate not only that the average American is 18 percent overweight but also that the incidence of obesity continues to increase. As a nation we are getting fatter, despite the plethora of weight control programs, diet books and increased emphasis on nutrition, physical fitness and health.

Every day millions of Americans go *on* diets and every day millions of Americans go *off* diets. People lose and people gain and round and round goes the vicious cycle. The overall failure rate in weight control is an alarming 95 percent; of those people who lose weight on a diet, only 5 percent will maintain their reduced weight for more than a year.

In the face of such overwhelming failure it is time that we stop blaming the overweight person for lack of motivation, willpower or what-have-you and start trying to find out why all the diets fail. It is time for a new attitude, a new approach and a totally new method of dieting. That is why this new fats reduction system presents such an exciting and welcome concept.

In physiological terms, the cure for obesity has been known for centuries. Just consume fewer calories than your body uses in a day. No magic, no mystery, just plain, well-known, well-established fact. Nearly all diets are designed to reduce calorie intake, nearly all can produce successful results. So why don't they?

The answers obviously lie in the vital psychological areas, and so often diet programs fail to take these into account. Most diets simply demand too much of normal human self-control. Sometimes they almost perversely seem to take away the very foods for which people most yearn, despite the fact that these foods, as in the case of many high carbohydrate foods for instance, are often far from being the most fattening foods.

As a psychiatrist I was delighted to discover the 7-Unit Low Fat Diet program presents a considerably less sacrificial way of reducing weight than previous dieting methods. Let me explain what I mean.

As well as eating to fill our stomachs, and supply our energy, we all have a deep psychological need to derive pleasure from the food we eat. If we don't feel that we have had our full quota of food for the day, in quantity, we tend to feel deprived. Strangely, at a more subconscious level, if we don't feel we have had our full pleasure quota of food for the day we also tend to feel deprived. That is one of the reasons why people who gobble down a meal mindlessly, while their minds are distracted by other things, often eat an additional meal later.

In order to gain maximum enjoyment from the food we eat, we need to be able to choose the foods we enjoy. Food preferences are highly individual. Diet programs that dictate exactly what we eat at each meal are rarely adhered to for long, for this reason. Freedom of food choice is essential and this new system provides a very wide area of freedom and flexibility.

In terms of the volume of food which can be eaten, this diet system has quite outstanding advantages. When we feel hungry we yearn for a good big meal. We don't yearn for "1,000 calories" or "1,500 calories"; what we want is good, tasty food and plenty of it. If we get that adequate quantity we will be satisfied and content whether the plateful provided just 400 calories or 1,400 calories. Our stomachs don't count calories as we eat!

Research in my feeding laboratory at the University of Pennsylvania, where I spent many years studying eating behavior, confirmed that this is true of people, and other research has even revealed that this concept is true of rats. Our short-term regulation of food intake is also governed by the volume of food consumed rather than by the number of calories consumed. In simple terms, if we get sufficient bulk of food we will be satisfied enough to stop eating, whether the calorie content of our meal is high or low.

Some foods can be eaten in very generous quantities at a very small cost in calories. Fruit and vegetables are prime examples. At the other end of the scale some foods give us only the most meager quantity for very high calorie cost. Fats are *the* outstanding example here.

In order to eat a generous quantity of food at a modest cost in calories it therefore makes total diet sense to reduce the foods that give us least for most calories—FATS!

Fats are by far the highest calorie foods in our diets. Consider for a moment that a single gram of butter, which is a minute quantity—about the size of one small pea—contains 7.2 calories.

A gram of corn, olive or peanut oil supplies a staggering 8.9 calories. You could pour 40 to 50 calories' worth of oil into one teaspoon!

By contrast, a gram of apple or orange supplies less than half a calorie so you would get a very reasonable sized slice, about one-fifth of the whole fruit, for the same calorie cost as that single pea-sized gram of butter.

In the past some dieting methods have been based on the severe restriction of carbohydrate foods, but this system has little real logic when you consider that even a gram of sugar (3.85 calories) provides less than half the calories of a gram of oil. Potatoes are much, much lower still, at .9 calories per gram. It is only when they are cooked in fat that they shoot up to nearly 6 calories a gram. The oil is adding no real volume to the quantity of potato you put on your plate but it is adding a vast number of calories.

You don't actually see that high-calorie fat when you eat a serving of French fried potatoes, and that is another reason why fat is such a dangerous and deceptive fattener. Its presence in food is often invisible. Butter melts into toast, oil disappears into salad, fats hide insidiously in meat. Therefore, not only are we deceived by the increased calories per volume of food, but psychologically we are tricked into consuming these unseen calories.

Another characteristic of fat is that it goes down easily, requiring little effort to swallow, as the phrase "melts in your mouth" suggests. My many years of work in the behavioral area of eating control leaves me in no doubt at all that this adds enormously to its fattening potential.

It is now a widely accepted general rule that the more quickly people eat, the more food they eat. Don't take my word for this— just look around next time you go into a restaurant and you will see the evidence for yourself. Almost invariably you will observe that the heavily overweight people are eating faster than the slim people.

The more slowly you eat, the less food you require to create a sense of satisfaction and eventual satiation. But fat can be eaten so rapidly that by the time your brain registers "enough" you may have gone way over your calorie quota for that meal—or that day—without even realizing it.

So fats are very fattening in a physiological sense, in that they are staggeringly high in calories, and also in a psychological sense in that they encourage us to eat vast quantities of calories that we hardly notice. Add to that the fact that there is growing concern about fat in relation to our health and general well-being.

The Select Committee on Nutrition and Human Needs of the U.S. Senate recognized the dangers in our overconsumption of fats when they drew up new dietary goals for Americans.

Refuting the claims of those who have been advising us to reduce carbohydrate intake, for our weight and health, they actually recommended an increase in the intake of sugar-free carbohydrate foods to the point where they account for a larger percentage of our total calorie intake.

But the goals stress that fat consumption should be reduced from the present approximate 40 percent of our total calorie intake to 30 percent, with even greater reduction of the saturated fats, supplied mainly by meats and dairy products, which have become so suspect in relation to heart disease.

Reduction of fat intake, by the method recommended in this book, achieves almost all the dietary goals recommended by the Senate committee. The new system in this book sets forth a plan for recognizing and keeping track of fat units: *no calorie counting, no giving up of favorite foods.* The limitation of fat will lead to a reduction of calories, a healthier diet and to weight loss.

After so many years and so many fad diets it is indeed heartening finally to have a system which addresses the major issues of permanent weight control: flexibility, lack of deprivation, freedom of food choice, reduction in calories and a healthier way of eating.

CHAPTER ONE

At Last—The Ideal
Weight Loss Diet

This book was published in England in 1979 under the title *Dieting Revolution*. It was immediately hailed as the first radically new approach to dieting in the last thirty years. It caught on with remarkable speed because it worked so well and produced astounding success in weight loss for so many people.

The diet was developed by the editors of Britain's *Slimming* magazine in consultation with nutritionists and physicians. The idea came from the realization that, while the dieting public was busy counting calories and carbohydrates—and having a tough time taking off weight—the experts (nutritionists and medical professionals) were trying a different method: reducing and controlling weight by cutting down on the visible and invisible fats. When they did that, the pounds dropped off and stayed off. The editors of *Slimming* were determined to find a way to take this method beyond the realm of the medical profession and adapt it for the general public.

THE FAT UNIT: THE DIET'S SECRET INGREDIENT

After much discussion and consultation, the British experts devised an entirely new measure of dieting, aptly called "the fat unit." A fat unit equals about 25 calories and 2.85 grams of fat.

and measures the total fat content of a food, including both saturated (mostly animal) and unsaturated fats (mostly vegetable). Fat is one of three vital nutrients found in all foods. The other two are protein and carbohydrates. But of these three, fat is the one most overweight people need to reduce in their diet, because fat is the most fattening of the three—about twice as likely to put fat on your body as either protein or carbohydrates.

Thus, the British discovered that if you restricted yourself to a certain number of fat units per day, *you could eat virtually anything else you wanted and still lose weight.* They settled on 10 fat units per day as the maximum daily allowance.

They found that their plan worked. People who followed the low fat diet easily lost weight without feeling hungry or deprived. However, there was an unusual complaint: many dieters wrote saying they had difficulty eating as many as 10 units of fat every day. Many said they were getting along just fine on only 7 fat units a day. Thus, in the American version of the book, we have lowered the allowed number of fat units to 7, in keeping with the British experience. This will allow you to lose weight even faster. A person on this diet is eating approximately 7 to 17 percent of his or her daily calories in fat, or fewer than 200 calories. In American terms, this is a very low fat diet.

That is the secret of this diet: a simple way to measure how much fat you're eating, so that you can eliminate much of it and also notice the fat disappearing from your body.

WHAT ABOUT SUGAR AND ALCOHOL?

You may be pleasantly surprised to learn that it's difficult to overdose on sweets without overdosing on fat (because most sugary foods are also high in fat, such as ice cream and cake). So, for most dieters on the 7-Unit Low Fat Diet, the sugar problem takes care of itself. Consequently, an overconsumption of non-fat sugary foods, such as sugary soft drinks, would retard weight loss and cut the effectiveness of the diet. To help the dieters for whom this is of concern, the London researchers devised what they call an "equivalent fat unit" for certain high sugar foods and alcoholic beverages. You will find a special food and beverage chart listing these "equivalent fat units" on pages 129–132. When following the diet, you must also include these "equivalent fat units" in your daily total.

The London researchers have also determined that a person who wishes may have one alcoholic drink a day, such as 12 ounces of beer, 4 ounces of wine, or one and a half ounces of distilled liquor, without damaging the diet, although weight loss will be faster without alcohol.

This book has been completely adapted for American dieters and contains everything you need to follow the diet: charts showing the number of fat units in more than 2,000 American foods, including many served at fast food chains, as well as low fat recipes, all brand new and strictly American.

Although the British jumped the gun on us with their low fat diet, they weren't alone in their research; we were just a length behind. American weight-loss experts have been using low fat diets in clinics and groups and have been conducting research on ways to devise a properly balanced diet with a minimum of fat. But the British got there first in one important way: they took the fat unit out of the laboratory and put it on paper into the hands of millions of readers who could comprehend it easily, and budget it into their diets. And the readers lost weight.

Now that this diet, with its foolproof fat-unit counting method, has reached the American public, it is being soundly applauded by the medical profession. It isn't gimmicky, it isn't trendy and it isn't a fad. It is based on common-sense eating. This is because it enhances your health instead of damaging it as some diets do, and it brings *lasting* weight loss through a change in eating habits. The only reason it hasn't been used widely before in this country is that nobody had devised a way to make fat counting so simple. Now this problem has been solved—and it is thoroughly explained in this book.

Dieters who have tried this method swear by it for three important reasons: they lose weight (and keep it off); they enjoy every meal and do not feel deprived, and the easy-to-follow meal plans and recipes in Part II make preparing meals a joy.

CHAPTER TWO

How We Tested the
New Low Fats System

BY DEREK MILLER

Derek Miller, lecturer in nutrition and leader of a research team at London University, is internationally recognized as one of the leading scientists researching into the problems of obesity. His scientific papers have revealed many new discoveries, particularly in the area of metabolism. He directed the team of dietitians and nutritionists who conducted the first trials into his new system of dieting.

In 1978 a group of overweight British women were assembled by myself and nutritionists from *Slimming* magazine, and were predictably startled to be given the kind of dieting advice that has never before been proffered to those embarking on a weight-reducing program.

They were told, for instance, that they could eat as much as they wished of foods like bread and potatoes. Foods that they had previously been taught to regard as "wickedly fattening."

Their aim was to shed weight. Our aim was to prove that a revolutionary new dieting system, which made total sense in theory, would actually work in reality when followed by normal overweight human beings.

Because fats contribute such a high percentage of calories to the average Western diet—around 40 percent—it made theoretical sense that reducing fat intake would be sufficient in itself to reduce calorie intake low enough to achieve a weight loss. Cut the fats and the calories will take care of themselves. We spent months working out a system by which it became possible and simple for any overweight person to reduce fat intake to the right level. Now we had to put it to the test.

Week by week we watched our dieters following their strange new rules with a growing sense of satisfaction from both their side and ours. By the end of the first month we were able to congratulate ourselves and announce triumphantly: It works!

Not only had they lost weight, but in many cases they had lost it at a much faster speed than would normally be expected on an average diet. One woman had actually lost 18½ pounds in just four weeks and several more had shed more than 15 surplus pounds during that period.

Examples of the speedy weight loss results achieved:

In a period of 4 weeks:
Mrs. H. Bennett, Chelsea, London, S.W.1.	18½ lbs.
Mrs. I. Colthart, South Harrow, Middlesex	11¼ lbs.
Mrs. M. Crowley, Hackney, London, E.5.	16 lbs.
Mrs. J. Khan, Cricklewood, London, N.W.2.	16½ lbs.
Miss G. Price, West Kensington, London, W.14.	17 lbs.

The reason for these speedy rates of weight loss was revealed later when we analyzed the eating records kept by each dieter. By strictly rationing fat intake to 10 units a day we had hoped that we would automatically ration calorie intake around the 1,500 calories on which the average dieter can shed surplus weight. What we discovered was that, by following the system, most dieters had actually reduced their calorie intake closer to 1,000 calories a day, thus achieving an even faster speed of weight loss.

During the following year, this revolutionary fat reducing system of dieting was put to an even greater test: the test of being tried by hundreds of thousands of dieters. When a booklet outlining the new system was put on sale throughout Britain by *Slimming* magazine, it achieved such explosive popularity that the magazine was forced to do continual reprints until they today have sold nearly a million copies. This is the kind of popularity and demand which arises only in those circumstances when people tell each other, "I've tried it, it works!"

This new system of dieting has now stood the test and established its popularity in Britain. And, because it isn't just a gimmick but a realistic method in line with modern and scientific discoveries, we believe it is here to stay as the diet of the future.

CHAPTER THREE

Why This Diet Works

FATTY FOODS ADD THE MOST WEIGHT

On the calorie scale, one ounce of butter is as fattening *as all the following foods put together:* a large carrot, a quarter-pound of mushrooms, a tomato, a green pepper, a large zucchini squash, a couple of asparagus spears, four radishes and an apple. The reason is that butter is 100 percent fat; *all* the calories in butter come from fat. The few calories in those other foods are nonfat calories.

A glance at any calorie chart will reveal that it is the *fat* in our diet—butter, margarine, cooking oil, meat fat—that is largely responsible for putting on weight. That's why you can quickly and easily lose weight—and keep it off—by doing only one thing: *restricting the amount of fat in your diet.* When you do that you automatically cut down on calories. Of course, you must be sure that in cutting down fat, your diet maintains the other ingredients you need.

All the highest calorie foods (those in the 200 calorie-an-ounce range) are fats. Ounce for ounce, they provide more than double the calories of even the very high carbohydrate foods like flour and sugar. And *all highest calorie foods* are fatty.

Those foods that rate in the region of 150 calories an ounce—chocolate, nuts, pastry, cream cheeses—all owe their high calories to their high fat content. You just can't have high calorie content in most foods without high fat.

Even the most modest quantity of fat contributes a remarkable and disproportionately high number of calories to any of the meals we eat. Thus, without appearing to overindulge, the average American consumes more than 40 percent of his or her daily calories in the form of fat.

POUNDS MELT AWAY

What would happen if you ate less fat? Simply, you would become slimmer. This is illustrated through studies of the eating habits of other countries that do not share our national weight problem.

In recent years nutritionists have found a direct parallel between the percentage of fats in national diets and the prevalence of weight problems. In Korea, where fats contribute only 8 percent to the average daily calorie intake, obesity is rare. In Japan, where a visitor's first major surprise could be the sight of some of the world's tiniest waistlines, the diet is based on low fat and fat-free foods such as fish and vegetables.

There's also evidence that increasing the proportion of complex carbohydrates in your menus—vegetables and grains—as recommended on this diet, may cause you to lose more weight, even though you eat the same number of calories. That surprising conclusion comes from a recent study on rats done by Dr. Patillo Donald and colleagues at the University of Virginia and reported in *Science* magazine, January 9, 1981. Scientists lowered the percentage of protein in the animals' diets at the same time as they raised the percentage of complex carbohydrates, and held the number of calories steady. Rats fed the higher percentage of carbohydrates and lower percentage of protein gained the least weight. For example, rats fed a diet of 25 percent protein, 10 percent fat and 65 percent complex carbohydrates gained one-fourth more weight than rats fed only 5 percent protein, 10 percent fat, and 85 percent complex carbohydrates. Animals fed only 2 percent protein, 10 percent fat and 88 percent complex carbohydrates *actually lost weight*—although they were eating the same number of calories as the rats that gained weight!

Scientists don't know why this happened. One theory is that the complex carbohydrates, being higher in fiber, may not be absorbed as readily into the body. In any event, Dr. Donald concluded that if you're trying to lose weight, you're better off to eat more complex carbohydrates and low amounts of fat and protein. Just as you will on this diet.

BALANCING THE SCALE—AND LOSING THE WEIGHT

All the surveys and all the calorie figures clearly point to one fact: it is the fats in our diet that are the major culprits. It is the fats that make us fat. Since that's the case, will reducing these foods, and *only* these foods, produce a sufficiently fast weight loss to satisfy the enthusiastic dieter? Even if that dieter continues to eat freely of foods like potatoes and pasta that are forbidden on many diets?

The answer is yes. Tests in Great Britain with overweight people who followed the low fat diet show that even when they were eating many other foods they were losing astounding amounts of weight. Some dieters lost as much as 7 pounds in a week and 30 pounds within two months—a remarkably rapid rate of weight loss. The results of their tests helped confirm the theory, already widely held by nutritional experts, that if fats are sufficiently reduced in the diet, it is extremely difficult to consume enough calories to remain overweight.

Stay within the 7-unit fat allowance and you will not have to cut down on anything else. That's the difference between good calories and bad ones.

COMMON SENSE AND THE 7-UNIT LOW FAT DIET

Fats and fatty foods have an extremely high caloric density. They provide a high number of calories in a small volume of food. To consume the same number of calories, while eating only fat-free or low fat foods, you would have to consume a huge volume of food—more than the average appetite could cope with.

The object of all dieting methods is to reduce the daily calorie requirement and to force the body to draw on its surplus store of fat. With the new 7-unit method of dieting, you can achieve this without weighing and calculating every item of food, as you must do when counting calories or carbohydrates.

Why have dieters had to wait this long to discover the easy fat-control method of dieting? Simply because fats, as noted, often are "invisible" in foods and meals and so usually are harder to spot than more obvious carbohydrates. Fats in large quantities can lurk in innocent-looking foods such as hard cheeses and lean meats. Without an expert guide such as this book provides, it is difficult to know how to avoid them or calculate how much of them you are ingesting.

FOLLOW OUR CHART

Our chart of basic and processed foods, our fat counter list, that follows later in this book (page 133), provides an easy-to-follow guide. You can use it to ration fats in your diet to the 7-unit level—the effective weight-loss level. We give a simple unit count to each listed food, based on the fat content of each. You are allowed 7 of these fat units a day. A high figure on the chart indicates a high fat (and, consequently, a high calorie) food. A low figure, like one-half or one unit, indicates a food you can eat, but with care within your daily 7 units. A zero figure indicates a food with negligible fat content, which means it is either very low in calories or would have to be eaten in unrealistically large quantities to interfere with weight loss.

Follow the simple rules of our fat unit charts and your scales will prove that you are automatically slashing your daily calorie intake. Just keep careful track of your fat units. Stick to the number 7 and the calories—and your weight loss—will take care of themselves. Of course, your doctor should be kept informed of your progress.

CHAPTER FOUR

How to Follow This Diet

There's only one rule to remember: Eat only 7 units of fat a day.

This book is your guide on how to do just that. As you read, you will learn:

- How to count fat units and stop at 7;
- How to plan ahead, so you don't use up all your fat unit allowance by lunchtime;
- What foods to avoid, which ones to go easy on, and which you can indulge in freely.

You will learn from the recipes and menus included in Part II how to eat well, even artistically, and with satisfaction. You will never leave the table feeling deprived.

Finally, you will learn from the extensive charts provided in Part III exactly how many units of fat are contained in almost every type of food and drink you might want to consume.

After a few days on this diet, the fat content of most items will become familiar to you; you won't have to look them up anymore. You will pick up the system quickly, and you'll learn the ropes: which foods use up more of your fat allowance than they're worth in terms of eating pleasure, such as avocados and

French fries (but we will show you in the recipe section how to make your own no-fat French fries, which you can eat freely), and which foods will give you a great deal of pleasure in return for the low number of fat units you spend on them (such as pasta and bread). You'll soon be budgeting your fat units as carefully as you budget your paycheck. And with the same happy results.

You'll find some surprises. So here is your first assignment: skim the charts in the back of this book. Make a note of any items in which fat content, or lack of it, surprises you. Pasta is a good example (see below).

One more assignment. Buy a pocket-size notebook, and use it to keep track of your daily expenditure of fat units. Consult it frequently. Are you spending your units wisely? If not, rethink your daily planning.

The aim of this diet is, of course, to lose weight. That's the aim of all weight loss diets. But the 7-Unit Low Fat Diet has another aim: to make eating pleasurable for you while you are losing weight. This is *not* a deprivation diet. You can be a gourmet—or a gourmand—as long as you *count those fat units*. The joy of this diet is that you can eat all the nonfat foods you want. Here are some of the advantages you will discover:

• If you have a passion for pasta, you can enjoy it frequently, as long as you are careful to inhibit oil, butter or other fatty substance in the sauce. (See page 000 for a super nonfat spaghetti sauce.)

• If you are fond of bread, you can eat almost all you want, although we wouldn't recommend that you use up all your units this way. Try, always, to vary your choice of foods both for good nutrition and for speedy weight loss. But bread is a "good" food and allowed on the 7-Unit Low Fat Diet.

• If red meat is your favorite food, you can eat a lean 8-ounce steak, a 5-ounce lean hamburger or even a McDonald's quarter-pounder daily!

• If you have a craving for sweets, you can have all the fresh fruits you want and you can include other sweet foods in your 7 units. But it's very likely that on this diet desire for empty calorie sweets will greatly diminish or disappear because you can eat other filling, comforting foods, such as sweet potatoes, spaghetti, hot breads, usually forbidden on other diets.

7 BASIC STEPS

In short, you can continue to indulge your own individual taste for food. Here is the simple, step-by-step daily program to follow. Seven steps, in fact, 7 *easy* steps. They are:

1. Figure out how many units of fat each food has before you eat it.

2. Plan your day's meals so that you will consume only 7 units of fat; budget carefully.

3. STOP when you reach the seventh unit. *That's all* the fat you can have for the day. You can, however, keep on enjoying other foods.

4. Keep a written record of your fat-unit intake. Over a period of weeks, or even days, you'll find yourself learning to plan more and more carefully. Some days you may even end up with a unit or more left over.

5. Analyze your mistakes (of course you'll make mistakes) and learn from them; make substitutions for foods that you know are not good fat-unit bargains.

6. Eat all you want of the foods that contain virtually no fat —pasta, grains, fresh fruit and vegetables—but *always* stop eating before you are full.

7. Be adventuresome! Try the recipes in this book, and follow the menus. Mix them up and improvise. Make your dieting experience a pleasurable one as well as a slimming one.

There you are: 7 steps, 7 units of fat, 7 days in the week to try new and different foods. It could be your lucky number—or your next clothing size.

CHAPTER FIVE

Three Capsule Lists to
Help You Follow the Diet

Before you proceed to the more comprehensive fat-unit charts at the end of this book, here are three capsule lists of foods you can eat when following this diet:
1. In *any* quantity.
2. In almost any quantity.
3. Very sparingly.

These minilists are easy to recall or to copy and carry with you.

1. FREE FOODS
Eat Without Restriction Until You Feel Satisfied*

These foods have no fat units:

---

* No foods are absolutely fat-free. Vegetables, including lettuce, have traces of fat. And a cup of cooked spaghetti has .7 grams. But the theory behind the diet is that these foods have so little fat compared with their ability to fill you up, that it would be difficult to consume enough of them to add significant amounts of weight. Thus, the designers of the diet assigned a 0 fat unit to such foods—usually those with .7 fat grams or fewer per serving. In some cases, also, the fat units have been adjusted to reflect the high sugar content of certain low fat foods, such as candied sweet potatoes and sweetened cereals, which would cause excessive weight gain, if eaten freely.

1. Bulgur wheat
2. Chestnuts
3. Condiments, made without oils, fats or egg yolks
4. Cottage cheese (uncreamed)
5. Crackers, fat free
6. Eggs (whites only)
7. Fresh fruits—all kinds
8. Milk (skim)
9. Pasta—macaroni, spaghetti, noodles
10. Rice
11. Spices, all kinds
12. Tea, coffee, diet soft drinks, club soda
13. Vegetables—all kinds except avocados, olives and certain beans, particularly soy beans
14. Yogurt (skim milk)

2. FAIRLY LOW-FAT FOODS
Eat Moderately

These foods have low to moderate numbers of fat units. You can eat them regularly, but keep track of their fat units by checking the food charts.

1. Bread of all kinds, rolls, plain muffins, tortillas
2. Cereals (see Fat Units Counter, page 146)
3. Cheeses (low fat)
4. Chicken, turkey without skin or fat, white meat preferred
5. Dried beans
6. Eggs (whole)
7. Fish
8. Meat (lean only)
9. Milk (low fat)
10. Nondairy creamers

11. Salad dressings (low fat)
12. Tuna (waterpacked)
13. Yogurt (low fat)

3. FOODS TO USE WITH CAUTION
Avoid—Or Eat Very Sparingly

1. Alcohol
2. Avocados, olives, soybeans
3. Butter, margarine, oils, salad dressing, mayonnaise, lard
4. Cakes, candy, sweetened gelatin
5. Cheese made from whole milk
6. Coconut
7. Cream and cream sauces
8. Dried fruits, sweetened canned fruits (low in fats but high in sugar)
9. Meats; fatty meats such as hot dogs, bacon, cold cuts, spareribs
10. Milk (whole)
11. Nuts, peanut butter
12. Potato chips
13. Soft drinks with sweeteners
14. Sour cream
15. Sugar, honey, molasses

CHAPTER SIX

Why This Diet Is Good for You

Which are the bad foods? None are really bad except when eaten in excess. But if you're like most Americans, you've grown up with the idea that meat and milk are wholesome and good for you, and potatoes, cereals, spaghetti are outrageously starchy and somehow bad for you. It is widely believed that they can manufacture fat faster than you can say their names. It's a commonly shared notion, but it's totally incorrect. Recently, government and medical authorities have been trying hard to erase that belief.

Excessive sugar is still regarded as detrimental to health, but recently there has been a decided shift to fats as dietary enemy number one. As Dr. Jordan observed in his Introduction to this book, Senator George McGovern's congressional subcommittee on nutrition pioneered in presenting evidence in 1977 that a high fat diet can contribute to illness and premature death.

Subsequently, agencies of the federal government concerned with nutrition have taken up the antifat campaign. The National Cancer Institute, the Surgeon General's Office, the Department of Health, Education and Welfare (now Department of Health and Human Services) and the U.S. Department of Agriculture all have recently issued major statements condemning fat, among other dietary factors.

In an unprecedented government action, HEW and USDA in February 1980, urged us to do the following to avoid excessive fat:

- Choose lean meat, fish, poultry, dry beans and peas as our protein sources.
- Moderate our use of eggs and organ meats.
- Limit our intake of butter, cream, hydrogenated margarines, shortenings and coconut oil, and foods made from such products.
- Trim excess fat off meats.
- Broil, bake or boil instead of fry.
- Read labels carefully to determine both the amount and types of fat contained in foods.

Nor is this country alone in its concern. Health officials in eight Western countries where diets are exceedingly high in fat have recommended cutting down on it.

Here are some of the dangers of a high fat diet:

- Fats, especially saturated fats (as found in meat and dairy products) can raise blood cholesterol. Thus, fatty foods are linked to heart disease and atherosclerosis.
- Fats displace more valuable foods in the diet, such as grain products, fruits and vegetables that provide roughage or fiber. (When you go on a low fat diet, you automatically increase your intake of fiber. Many experts think fiber helps prevent digestive diseases, colon cancer and possibly other diseases.)
- Fats in foods are the depositories for many pesticides and other dangerous chemicals in the environment. Cutting down on fats reduces your exposure to such chemicals.
- Fats—both saturated (primarily in meat and dairy products) and unsaturated (mainly in vegetable products)—are increasingly being linked with cancer, especially of the breast and colon. Too much fat is thought to "promote" the growth of cancer.
- Fats may be a culprit in many other kinds of diseases, according to recent research. For example, women on a high fat

diet, according to one study, were more likely to develop toxemia during pregnancy, which can cause loss of the fetus or the mother's death.

- Fats, of course, are a primary cause of overweight, a condition that increases your risk of cardiovascular disease, high blood pressure, diabetes mellitus, hernia, gallbladder and liver diseases.

What is the ideal diet then? The Senate committee made these recommendations:

1. Increase your use of fruits and vegetables and whole grains.

2. Decrease your use of meat and increase consumption of poultry and fish.

3. Decrease your use of foods high in fat and partially substitute polyunsaturated fat for saturated fat.

4. Substitute skim or low fat milk for whole milk.

5. Decrease your use of butterfat, eggs and other high cholesterol sources.

6. Decrease your use of sugar and foods high in sugar content.

7. Decrease your use of salt and foods high in salt content.

The new 7-Unit Low Fat Diet does all of these things except the last, but if you want, you can do that too.

When you go on this diet, you automatically follow the same pattern as the one most highly recommended for your health.

- Since this diet is low in fat content, it inevitably is also a cholesterol-lowering diet.
- This diet is generous with grain products: cereals, rice, bread, pasta.
- This diet restricts the use of meat, which is high in fat, and encourages you to eat more chicken and fish which are lower in fat.
- This diet is low in sugar content. As noted, most foods high in sugar also tend to be high in fat. Cakes, chocolate, cookies are typical examples. Thus, by avoiding them because of their fat, you also cut out unwanted sugar. Also, in

cases where you might overindulge in sweet high-calorie foods, we have established equivalent fat units to help you keep sugar under control.

• This diet is generous with fruit and vegetables of all kinds. They can be eaten in unlimited quantities—except for avocado, which is extraordinarily fatty. The modest amount of sugar that occurs naturally in fresh fruit is not considered by experts to be damaging to your health.

The 7-Unit Low Fat Diet *will not leave you feeling constantly hungry,* as many diets do, because you can eat foods like potatoes, bread and spaghetti that make you feel full.

THE 7-UNIT LOW FAT DIET PROVIDES ALL THE PROTEIN AND OTHER NUTRIENTS YOU NEED

To be at optimum health, you must be sure to get enough protein. In this country, that's usually a needless warning. Most of us suffer from the *opposite* condition: consuming far more protein than we need.

However, many of our high fat foods are also our high protein foods; for example, whole milk, cheeses, red meats. On this diet you will be cutting down on high fat foods, which could mean automatically cutting down on some high protein sources. It is essential on any diet to get enough protein. But that will not be a problem on this diet because you can easily substitute foods that are low in fat and high in protein. In fact, you probably will do it automatically.

One of the best ways to get high protein along with low fat is to substitute the nonfat dry milk, low fat, or skim milk for whole milk, and use uncreamed instead of creamed cottage cheese. Chicken and fish also yield more protein per fat unit than red meats. Low fat fried beans, which can be cooked in a variety of delicious ways, are an *excellent* source of protein.

This chart shows some of the best low fat, high protein foods, and how much of your daily protein requirements they supply:

Food	Fat Units	Percentage of Daily Protein Requirement
Nonfat dry milk: ½ cup	0	50
Evaporated skim milk: 1 cup	0	40
Skim milk: 1 cup	0	40
Buttermilk, skim: 1 cup	0	20
Cottage cheese, dry, un-creamed: 1 cup	½	80
Yogurt: 8 oz.	½	25
Dried beans or other lentils; cooked: 1 cup	½	35
Tuna in water: 3 oz.	1	50
Chicken, roasted, without skin: 3½ oz.	3	50
Ground beef, lean, broiled: 3 oz.	3	50

THE IMPORTANCE OF OTHER NUTRIENTS

Increasingly researchers are finding that trace minerals—minute amounts of minerals in all kinds of foods—are essential and that trace-mineral deprivation could be dangerous in numerous ways. Grains, allowed freely on this diet, are an important source of trace minerals. But some grain products are more beneficial than others, especially when restricting your food intake. It is far wiser to eat whole grain foods to help ensure you're getting all the nutrients—mainly trace minerals—you need.

Here are some suggestions for the wise use of your fat units on this diet:

- When possible, choose whole grain breads over white bread; the flour used in the latter has been stripped of many nutrients during processing.
- Pasta, which you can eat freely, is generally made from white enriched flour, but some stores now offer whole wheat pasta, which is heavier in texture, but more nutritious. Try

it. If it's not in your supermarket, look for it in a health food store or an Italian grocery.

- Brown rice, which still retains the husk and natural nutrients, is preferable to white rice.
- Whole grain cereals, such as brans, Shredded Wheat, Grape Nuts, are more nutritious than modern processed cereals, often made from white flour.

These whole grain foods also contain much more fiber, which nutritionists increasingly believe is essential to maintaining health, preventing diseases, and promoting weight loss.

DO VITAMINS HELP?

It also doesn't hurt to take a multiple-vitamin mineral supplement daily as insurance. Some doctors call vitamin mineral supplements a waste of money and unnecessary, but many experts are now changing their minds about that. They realize that it's difficult to get all the vitamins and minerals you need from food —especially if you're cutting back on some foods to lose weight. There's also a growing body of evidence that larger doses of vitamins and minerals may protect some persons against disease. Supplements are no substitute for food, however, and the best policy is to eat a variety of foods, especially the vitamin and mineral rich grains, vegetables and fruits which are the foundation of the 7-Unit Low Fat Diet. But a vitamin mineral supplement can give added protection.

CHAPTER SEVEN

The 7-Unit Low Fat Diet
Is Not a Fad Diet

So much nonsense has been written about dieting in recent years (often, sadly, by doctors) that we want you to realize you are not being misled again.

Many such books and diets suggest that certain foods have special chemical (or magical) qualities which enable them to melt away body fat or, on the other hand, to relentlessly add to body fat. We all remember, for instance, the grapefruit diet, and its implication that grapefruit possessed some special body-fat melting qualities. If only it did!

Worse was the so-called diet that advocated eating high amounts of fat to lose weight.

The reason some of these nonsense diets work is that they reduce the total number of calories consumed in a day. Because of this some people succeed in losing weight. They then believe they have lost weight because they have been eating grapefruits or consuming the right amount of some other substance, and so the word spreads. In fact, they have dropped weight simply because they have reduced their overall calorie intake.

So let us make clear what the 7-Unit Low Fat Diet will accomplish. This new fat-unit system is designed to provide an easier, healthful way to reduce your total calorie intake sufficiently so that you lose surplus weight.

Cutting calories is what weight loss is all about. Cutting out fats is the supreme way of cutting out calories.

WHY FAT COUNTING CAN BEAT CALORIE COUNTING

The big drawback of the calorie-counting system of dieting is the work involved. For some people the discipline of weighing and counting every item of food consumed proves to be too much effort. The low fat unit diet is much simpler. All the fat-free foods can be eaten in any quantity without being weighed or calculated. Those containing fat are given a simple unit count so that you only have to add up to 7 each day—and stop counting there. There is no need to calculate every bite you put in your mouth.

WHY FAT COUNTING CAN BEAT CARBOHYDRATE COUNTING

The low carbohydrate diet has been one of the most popular ways of losing weight in the last two decades. The new low fat unit method of dieting is as easy as counting carbohydrates in that only certain foods must be restricted while others can be eaten freely. Where the two diets differ vastly is in the types of foods which are restricted.

Dieting likes and dislikes differ. For some people the low carbohydrate method—which rations only sweet and starchy foods —has proved an effective way to lose weight. But here are the definite advantages to the low fat method.

SURER WEIGHT REDUCTION

If you cut out most of the sugary and starchy foods from your diet by counting carbohydrates, you will eliminate many high calorie foods (carbohydrates are often combined with fats in foods like cakes, pastries, cookies, chocolate). Generally, you will also tend to eat less. As a result, you should reduce your calorie intake sufficiently to lose weight.

However, some potentially highly fattening foods, such as heavily marbled meats, butter, cheeses, are negligible in carbohydrate content. And by eating them freely—as the low carbohydrate diet allows you to do—you can inadvertently slow or even stop your weight loss, particularly in the latter stages of your diet.

All diets work by reducing overall calorie intake. Unfortunately, the quantity of carbohydrate supplied by a particular food does not necessarily bear a direct relationship to its calorie content or, thus, to its fattening potential. For example, pure fats such as butter, margarine, cooking oil, lard, the most fattening foods of all, are not limited in the low carbohydrate diet. By taking the "no restrictions" advice too literally and eating foods with a liberal quantity of fat, some low carbohydrate dieters inadvertently slow their weight loss.

The same could happen with an overindulgence in high protein foods on the low carbohydrate diet. Foods high in protein vary a great deal in caloric content—from just over a modest 20 calories an ounce for grilled white fish to about 120 highly concentrated calories an ounce for some hard cheeses. The low carbohydrate diet takes no account of these variations, because meat, fish, cheese and eggs—all foods high in protein—are negligible in carbohydrates. Again it is possible to retard your weight loss by indulging in large quantities of high-calorie high protein foods.

One of the greatest inconsistencies of the low carbohydrate diet is that cream is often unrestricted because of its negligible carbohydrate content, while lower-calorie milk, which does contain carbohydrate, is limited. In fact, heavy cream supplies almost *thirteen times* the calories of an equal quantity of skimmed milk and therefore is *much* more fattening.

In contrast, the fat content of any food bears a *direct* relationship to its calorie content. *All* high fat foods are high calorie foods. Thus, on the 7-Unit Low Fat Diet you will eat high protein foods that do not add excessive calories. You simply find the safest protein foods by consulting the Fat Units chart (page 133). You will find that high calorie protein-containing foods, such as hard cheeses and fatty meats, automatically have a higher fat unit count than potentially less fattening protein foods—for example, chicken, fish, yogurt and dry cottage cheese, skim or nonfat dry milk. And you select the best high protein but low fat bargain. *The Fat Units chart provides a safer method of ensuring that you do not exceed the calorie limit necessary to maintain a good rate of weight loss or weight control, once you've lost enough to reach your goal.*

LOWER CALORIE INTAKE

By following the low fat method of dieting you will consume fewer calories than by following a low carbohydrate method, and lose weight faster. The fewer calories you consume, the more quickly you shed pounds.

Because of the lack of restriction of certain high calorie foods, in particular fats and high calorie protein foods, the average low carbohydrate dieter often consumes at least 1,500 calories a day. This tends to be the maximum level at which a satisfactory weight loss can be achieved. For some people—in particular those who are only a little overweight and who have been dieting a long time—1,500 calories may be too many to produce weight loss.

But the low fat method automatically limits *all* the very highest calorie foods. On this diet you will naturally direct your choice of protein-containing foods to the lower fat ones that are a better diet bargain, so you will be taking in *fewer* calories for the *same or more* quantity of protein-bearing foods.

An analysis of the diets of our test-team dieters who followed the low fat unit diet showed the average dieter was consuming slightly under 1,000 calories a day. This makes the low fat diet method especially suitable for those aiming to lose weight quickly or those who need to ration their calorie intake to lower than average dieting level in order to achieve a satisfactory weight loss.

YOU CAN EAT MORE FRUITS AND VEGETABLES

On the 7-Unit Low Fat Diet you can freely eat most fruits and vegetables without fear of gaining weight. Unfortunately, because of the lack of direct relationship between calorie and carbohydrate content, all fresh fruit and some vegetables are limited to an extreme and unnecessary degree on the low carbohydrate method of dieting.

An apple, orange or pear, for instance, will cost 2 of your 10 daily carbohydrate units on such a diet. This is too expensive a price to pay because each piece of fruit supplies only around 40 calories—a very modest bite out of a dieter's allowance of 1,000 to 1,500 calories a day. Furthermore, many dieters, who are not allowed to fill up with salads, fruit and vegetables on this diet, find themselves constantly hungry for more bulk in their stomachs.

The foods any person on the 7-Unit Low Fat Diet can afford to eat with most freedom are fresh fruit and vegetables—all vegetables as long as they are cooked and served without fat, even potatoes, which supply only 25 calories an ounce!

CHAPTER EIGHT

The 7-Unit Low Fat Diet
Will Save You Money, Too!

You don't have to buy a lot of fancy foods to go on this diet. In fact, most of the foods you will eat are among the least expensive you can find. The diet not only fights fat, it also fights inflation.

Ironically, fat is expensive, one of the most expensive ingredients in our diet. For example, the better marbled a steak—the more fat it contains—the higher its price. Our milk is even priced according to its fat content—the greater the percentage of fat, the higher its value. It has long been a badge of affluence for Americans to eat a lot of high fat foods and to look down on the lower cost diets of dried beans, rice, vegetables, chicken and fish, bread and potatoes, common in South American, Eastern European, Asian and Third World diets. But now nutritional experts are realizing that our extravagance—our premium on fat—is foolish: a waste of money and dangerous to our health. Consistently, in countries where the diets are simpler and less rich, there is a lower rate of chronic diseases such as atherosclerosis and heart disease. (For a more thorough discussion, see Afterword, page 189.)

Nutritional thinking in this country is undergoing a big turnabout. You may have noticed, for example, that the trend to cut down on meat, even to the point of adopting vegetarianism, is becoming more popular. The late anthropologist Margaret Mead predicted that within fifty years the United States would be largely vegetarian, mainly because it will be cheaper in the long run to feed ourselves on vegetables and grains and better for our health. Our high fat diets are becoming ever more expensive to maintain. Which is why, on the frontiers of nutrition, high priced, high fat, Western-style diets are fading and low cost, low fat "peasant" foods are coming in.

Here's how you'll be saving money on this diet:

You'll be eating more poultry, which is cheaper than red meats.

You'll be eating fewer convenience foods that are higher in price because the cost of packaging and preparation must be figured into their sales price.

You'll be eating more dried beans as a protein source, instead of expensive meats.

You'll be cutting back on expensive processed meats, such as hot dogs and bacon, which are very high in fat.

You'll be eating more rice, potatoes and bread, which are traditionally less expensive and give you more bulk for the dollar.

You'll be cutting back on expensive butter, cheeses and margarine.

So you'll be cutting dollars off your grocery bill at the same time you trim pounds off your figure!

CHAPTER NINE

Tips on Eating Out

Restaurant chefs, just as you do, make their dishes from a combination of a few basic foods: that is true the world over. No matter how exotic the concoction, it is still made from a small number of basic foods that fall into distinct groups: dairy products (milk, cream, cheese, butter); grain products (rice, pasta, bread, cereals); vegetables and fruits; animal meats (chicken, seafood, red meats); eggs and nuts. Some are fatty; some are not.

Once you are familiar with the fat units in a few basic foods, you will have little difficulty dining out on this diet. In fact, it can be fun.

Here are some suggestions:

1. *Vegetables and fruits.* Plain. Sure bets—any meal, any time of day (except avocado and coconut). Ask that sauces and butter be left off. Sauces are almost sure to be made from cream, butter and/or meat fats or oils, and loaded with fat units.

Baked potatoes, available in many restaurants, are an ideal eat-out food; they are a wonderful, filling food with great texture and taste. Many of us have forgotten how good they can be plain because we're so used to dousing them with sour cream and butter. For extra flavor, try topping them with nonfat sauces, such as Worcestershire sauce or other vegetables, for example, chopped onions. A baked potato topped with sauerkraut is an excellent combination.

If platters come with French fries, ask that they be left off. See if you can get a substitute of a baked potato or plain vegetable or salad.

All kinds of fruit and vegetable salads are good bets for low fat eating out. They usually have no fat units until you add a dressing; request yours served without dressing. On the traditional Chef's Salad, ask that the cheese and ham be left off. Ask for chicken or turkey instead. Ham, salami and other cold cuts that sometimes show up on such salads are higher in fat. Ask to mix the oil and vinegar dressing yourself, so you can control the amount of fatty oil if you want it. Or better yet, ask for fresh lemon to squeeze on the salad. Use nonfat cocktail sauce, instead of mayonnaise or tartar sauce, on salads containing meat or seafood.

2. *Grain products.* Any restaurant has cereals, and those—either hot or cold—are an excellent way to start the day. Spare the sugar and avoid presweetened cereals (remember, sugar counts as an equivalent fat unit). For a bit of sweetness try plain fruits: bananas, apples, pears, berries. Use nonfat skim or low fat milk.

Remember, you can eat bread, which you'll never find lacking in restaurants. Each one-ounce slice of any kind—white, whole wheat, sour dough, rye, muffins—only counts for one-half a fat unit. Just ask that it come without butter or any kind of grilling that could add oil.

Rice is another filling food you can eat plenty of, as long as it's not doused with butter, gravy or rich sauces. Rice is one of the things that makes Chinese restaurants appealing on this diet. Orientals generally are known for their low fat cooking. They do use vegetable oils, but rarely very much, and often make sauces and soups from low fat broths instead of meat and dairy fats. Generally, many of the meats in Oriental restaurants are grilled and are served with nonfat or low fat sauces, based on soy sauce. (Soy sauce, however, is very high in salt, and should be restricted by people with high blood pressure; too much sodium can aggravate the condition.)

The clear broth soups, rice and abundance of vegetables make Oriental cooking a good choice on this diet. However, some notable high fat foods to avoid are: deep-fried batter-covered seafood and poultry, egg rolls, crunchy chow mein noodles and sweet and sour dishes that are often loaded with sugar.

Spaghetti, macaroni, noodles are all good on this diet, as long as they're not drenched in fat-based sauces. Although it's difficult to convince people of this, a plate of spaghetti with a low fat sauce—for example, a plain tomato or marinara sauce without meat—is an excellent diet dish. The fact that you come away feeling full doesn't mean you're doomed to put on weight. On this diet you don't have to go around feeling hungry all the time, because many of the low fat foods are the most filling—bread, potatoes, pasta.

Italian restaurants are just fine, if you stick to plain sauces, don't sprinkle on cheese or order dishes heavy in cheese, cream or meat sauces. Fettucine Alfredo—with butter and cream sauce —is not a low fat diet food. On the other hand, plain spaghetti and tomato sauce is. Although every restaurant has its own recipe, it is generally safe to count 2 fat units for every half-cup of tomato sauce when eating out.

3. *Meats, poultry and seafood.* Choose plain broiled or baked chicken, roasts and broiled meats and broiled seafood instead of dishes swimming in butter or oil. Ask the waiter to leave off such sauces, or at least to serve them on the side. Avoid deep-fried seafood, such as shrimp and fish. When ordering chicken or poultry, remove the skin before eating. With red meats, cut off all the visible fat if the chef hasn't done it for you. This will go a long way toward getting rid of the fat in red meats, such as beef, lamb and pork. Even so, red meats are still higher in fat units than chicken and seafood.

Go easy on processed meats such as pastrami, hot dogs, bologna, bacon and cold cuts, which are often about 80 percent fat. If you must eat bacon, choose Canadian bacon, which is much leaner and lower in fat.

Best bet is a chicken or turkey sandwich (hold the mayonnaise; try lettuce and tomato instead). Plain canned tunafish, often found on restaurant salad platters, is also low in fat units. Best of all, ask if the restaurant has tunafish packed in water.

Hamburgers, except in very high class restaurants, are generally fatty and greasy. If you do order a hamburger or other meat where grease is visible, blot the grease off with a paper napkin. Also, hamburgers ordered well done have more of the fat cooked out.

Meat salad sandwiches, such as ham salad, made with mayonnaise, are not good foods on this diet. One tablespoon of mayonnaise will cost you 4 of your daily 7 fat units.

4. *Dairy products.* These are usually the nemesis of a low fat dieter. In restaurants, you can avoid whole milks, cream, butter and most hard cheeses. Cottage cheese is excellent (most restaurants have it) and many restaurants now stock low fat or skim milk. Ask for it; if more people do, more restaurants will start to use it.

5. *Eggs.* If you eat eggs out, ask for hard-boiled or poached to avoid the extra fat.

Some do's and don'ts when eating out on this diet:

- Use lemon or vinegar on salads, or ask for low calorie, low fat salad dressings.
- Avoid dishes with butter and cream sauces and gravies which are almost sure to be high fat.
- Ask for skim milk instead of whole milk.
- Ask for fish and meat broiled without oil or butter.
- Avoid sour cream.
- Forgo butter, margarine and mayonnaise.
- Cut all visible fat off meat. If you can't avoid deep-fried, battered foods, remove the crust before eating.
- Forgo heavy desserts made with cream, chocolate and sugar.

EATING OUT BASIC FOOD CHART

In the beginning, you may want to copy out and carry with you this list of the fat units in basic foods, until you are familiar with them. For fast foods, such as Big Macs, you can consult the brand name list in this book (page 184).

Dairy products and eggs	*Fat Units*
Milk, whole: 1 cup	3
Milk, skim: 1 cup	0
Cream, heavy: 1 tbsp	2
Cheese, hard: 1 oz. (1-inch cube)	3
Cottage cheese, dry or low fat: 1 cup	1
Butter: 1 tbsp	4
Yogurt, low fat: 1 cup (without fruit)	½
Eggs, whole: 1 egg	2

Grain products	
Bread: 1 slice or one muffin or 1 oz.	½
Cereal, without sugar: 1 oz.	½
Rice, spaghetti, macaroni, bulgur wheat, all other grains, plain	0

Meats	
Beef: 3 oz. lean	3
Chicken, no skin, roasted: 3 oz. white meat	1½
Fish, plain (most types): 3 oz.	½
Shellfish: 3 oz.	½

Fruits and vegetables	
All fresh vegetables (except avocados and soybeans)	0
All fresh fruits (except coconut)	0

Oils	
Margarine: 1 tbsp	4
Mayonnaise: 1 tbsp	4
Salad dressings: regular: 1 tbsp	2½
diet, low fat, low calorie: 1 tbsp	½

Beverages (equivalent fat units)	
Soft drinks containing sugar: 8 fl. oz.	4
Soft drinks, low or no calorie	0

	Fat Units
Coffee, tea	0
Alcohol: 1½ fl. oz.	4 (average)
Beer: regular: 12 fl. oz.	6
light: 12 fl. oz.	4
Wine: dry: 1 fl. oz.	1

CHAPTER TEN

Here's How to *Stay* Thin

After you reach your desired weight, if you want to splurge a little all you need do is to slightly increase the number of fat units you eat a day. Experiment by adding 5 or more fat units per day—and you will quickly find how many you can tolerate and still keep your weight steady if you weigh daily at the same time and under the same circumstances.

One of the most exciting facts emerging from experience with this diet is that on it you can easily manage to keep your weight down without the agony of having to give up forever some of your favorite foods.

Few of us are capable of making eternal sacrifices at the table. Having become slim by the fat unit counting method, you almost certainly will want to eat some of your favorite foods, even if they have a high fat content.

However, once you become aware of the enormous weight-producing potential of fats, as you will by following this diet, you will also realize that you were inadvertently consuming more fatty calories than you really wanted or needed. You will discover that there are ways to cut down on fats without making a real sacrifice.

In the future we suspect you will automatically use a little less butter in gravy, scrambled eggs, mashed potatoes and casseroles. You will find yourself eating more chicken and fewer delicatessen meats and hot dogs. Using low fat or skim milk instead of whole milk. Eating more sherbet and less rich ice cream.

When you come to realize how fattening fat really is—and how easy it is to cut out much of the excess—you will then effortlessly develop new eating patterns that enable you to remain thin.

CHAPTER ELEVEN

What Happy Dieters Have to Say

When *Slimming* magazine published the Low Fat Diet, as we told you at the beginning of the book, they were deluged with mail. We thought you'd be interested in what these Englishwomen found out about the low fat way of losing weight.

> I have been on your low fat unit diet for five weeks and am absolutely thrilled to say that I have lost 27 pounds.
> The diet sounded too good to be true, but I thought I would give it a trial, and this is the result. Over the years we have been so conditioned not to eat many of the free foods mentioned that one cannot believe you can eat them and still lose weight. Well, I have proved that you can.
>
> (Mrs.) A.R.K.

> I am a married woman with two small sons. I am 28 years old. I had tried dozens of diets and even went into the hospital for five weeks on a starvation diet, but nothing ever really happened. I lost quite a few pounds, but then drifted back because the diets were such a bore to me. Then came your low fat diet. Now after only one week I have lost seven pounds. I really enjoy dieting

now. I feel happier and ready to lose weight. I want to get down to 170 pounds, and I believe that on this diet I can do it.

I want to thank you from the bottom of my heart for showing me the best and easiest diet I have ever had.

(Mrs.) J.K.

P.S. Plus this is the first diet that really fits in with the family.

From April 10 to August 30 I have now lost a total of 42 pounds on the low fat diet. I feel this is a real breakthrough for people like me who have struggled with a weight problem for years.

(Mrs.) A.A.

I have always had a weight problem. I was overweight as a child; when I started work in 1953 I was over 168 pounds. Soon I was nearly 190 pounds, and was given a 1,000-calorie diet by the endocrinologist at the hospital I was working for. I reduced to about 120, but soon started creeping back up. By 1966 I was over 200 pounds and decided to reduce again, this time I did it much more slowly, but again by keeping a check on calories. I got down to 130 pounds and remained at this for some years. I knew it was not as low as I should go for my height of 5′ 2″, but it was a great achievement to me to be able to maintain that weight.

Then since 1976 weight had crept up again to nearly 170 pounds. Last year I managed to lose around 15 pounds, but put some of it back on again.

Now comes the best part. Since February (five months) I have reduced from over 155 pounds to 137. I find the new low fat diet marvellous. It's much easier to count fat units instead of calories. I quickly learned all the foods which are rated at "0," and eat a lot of toast and fruit and use skim milk all the time instead of ordinary milk.

The big advantage with this diet is that I am never hungry (when I counted calories I nearly always felt hungry) because I can have more carbohydrates. I think it is a much better way of eating and I am sure it will be easier to adjust to a maintenance diet when I again reach 130 pounds.

(Mrs.) J.M.W.

I just wanted to let you know that I have been on your diet for two weeks and have lost seven pounds with little effort. I have tried diets before but have always found them very hard to stick to. This new low fat diet of yours does appear to be the answer.

(Mrs.) L.F.

As someone who has been trying to lose weight for some years— unsuccessfully—I have found your low fat diet very good. I can now diet without cooking separate meals for myself. As a mother of two and working full time I find it very difficult to work out calories and carbohydrates when preparing meals.

(Mrs.) J.C.

At last a diet I enjoy and don't feel ravenous on. I have been on it two weeks and have lost 12 pounds. I was 181 pounds and only five feet four.

(Mrs.) T.R.

May I tell you how delighted I am with the success of the low fat dieting method. Since commencing on January 24 (seven months ago) I have shed 22 pounds. During this time not once have I suffered the pangs of unsatisfied hunger.

I must hasten to add that during my dieting period I spent a week in Italy in which time I restricted myself not one iota, so you can see that my weight loss is even more remarkable.

Several times in the past I have shed weight by painful methods, only to find it creeping back in due course. This time, I am firmly convinced that with your method—in the future I shall have no problem ever again.

(Mr.) B.M.

Low fat dieting is not like any dieting I've done before. Of course, there are still some much-loved foods I've had to give up, like cheesecake and fried onions, but this is almost over- compensated for by the fact that I don't have to restrict eating bread, potatoes and spaghetti with tomato sauce (a favorite).

Needless to say, I've started losing weight and have made a graph to measure my weight loss. After the first week I lost four pounds. I was thrilled to bits. When I was on a calorie-controlled diet, I remember it being really hard going and it obviously didn't change my eating pattern for the long term.

(Mrs.) M.S.

Here I am again to tell you about my fantastic success with your low fat diet. In the first week I dropped from 126 pounds to 119 pounds, and one week later I'm now 116 pounds. I haven't felt hungry. I vary the diet every day and feel twice as energetic as I did. I've told so many people about this diet (because its success is so obvious) that I feel the whole population of Bristol must be on this diet.

L.W.

Your low fat diet is just what I have been looking for in a diet. I don't feel hungry, knowing that I can eat virtually anything even after I've counted my fat units.

Although I have only been on this diet for two weeks, I have lost 7 pounds off my 143 pounds. I am seventeen.

N.S.

Great! I think I have found (after 23 years of misery) *the* diet. I really think I can do it on your new "Low Fat Diet" method. I have just eaten my first meal—two rounds of slimming bread topped with a dish of spaghetti—and I feel full. And I didn't miss the butter. I'm really excited and feel I have a *real* chance this time!

(Mrs.) R.M.

Since the age of twenty-one, and especially after my two children —now aged twelve and eleven, came along I have had a constant weight problem.

Over the past ten years I have fluctuated between a size 12 and a size 18. But keeping below a size 18 was always a constant battle. I have tried crash diets, vigorous exercises, long walks, many different forms of slimming tablets, eating bananas and drinking milk only each day. I even tried sleeping in a polyethylene bag for several nights! Some of these methods worked for a while but all of them had side effects. If I wasn't exhausted all day, I was irritable and very depressed.

Exactly a month ago and almost into a size 18 I decided to give up any more attempts to lose weight. "The battle is over," I announced to my family. We would all have to accept that I would be fat and forty just like my twin sister and my mother's side of the family.

I cannot tell you how miserable I was. One afternoon, however, I caught sight of your book on the counter of the local paper shop. At first I was not at all convinced that eating as many potatoes and other starches as I wanted, despite counting fat units, could ever work. I therefore didn't announce to my family that I was dieting yet again! I cut out butter immediately and always took silent note of all the other foods you list containing fat units, making sure I never ate them in excess. My dieting went unnoticed! I piled my plate high at each meal with potatoes, rice or veg and I took piles of sandwiches for my lunch at the office, containing no butter or margarine, but heaped with filling containing no fat units. That was a month ago! I have never been irritable or hungry and I feel fit and well. And I am 19 pounds lighter!

When I was able to wear a size 14 pair of slacks to the office this morning, I decided to send you this letter.

(Mrs.) T.M.

With the help of the low fat diet I have lost 35 pounds. I saw the book in a newsagent's while buying birthday cards and thought I would give it a try. I weighed 150 pounds and at five feet two inches, you can imagine the rest. We breed horses, and do a lot of showing "in hand" (running the horse, not riding). You can imagine what my bottom looked like last year! I got to the stage where I hated to show the horses. But this year I have had no embarrassing moments, and know that the judges are watching the horse and not my fat bottom wobbling up and down.

(Mrs.) S.B.

I have found the diet extremely helpful in my "battle of the bulge." It is the very first dietary advice I have ever had no hesitation in recommending to friends.

I have lost a fair amount of weight with hardly any effort at all.

(Mrs.) T.H.

PART II

THE 7-UNIT LOW FAT DIET

Menu and Recipe Section

21 Tips for Low Fat Cooking

Cooking methods can, of course, dramatically affect your fat unit diet.

So here we list important dos and don'ts in low fat cooking, and give a variety of fat unit counted recipes of appetizing dishes cooked in the least fattening way.

1. Roast meat and poultry on a rack so they do not sit in the fat in the roasting pan. Do not baste during cooking.

2. Poach eggs in simmering water with a dash of vinegar. Do not use a greased poacher.

3. Cornstarch can be substituted for arrowroot: 2 tablespoons arrowroot equals 1 tablespoon cornstarch. Cornstarch must be mixed with a small amount of water or other liquid before blending it with other ingredients.

4. Make a gravy from a stock cube and water thickened with a little cornstarch. Do not use the fatty meat juices in the roasting pan.

5. Do not brush foods with oil or fat before broiling.

6. Cut off all visible fat from meat.

7. Fat can be removed from a casserole by cooling the dish

quickly when cooked. Lift the set fat off the surface. Reheat very thoroughly before eating. If the casserole is needed immediately, mop up any fat globules on the surface with a paper towel.

8. Brown chopped beef in a nonstick pan before using and carefully drain off all the fat.

9. Do not fry meat or vegetables before making a stew or casserole. It is not necessary and will result in no loss of flavor.

10. Remove all skin from chicken and turkey before eating.

11. Drain all oil from canned tuna and sardines before using and strain in a colander under water. Mop up any excess oil with paper towels.

12. Make homemade soups by simmering vegetables in stock or water and then sifting or blending in a food processor. To thicken when reheating, add a little powdered skimmed milk or cornstarch.

13. Use skimmed or low fat milk instead of ordinary milk in recipes.

14. Use yogurt seasoned with salt and pepper as a delicious salad dressing.

15. Make stock from a stock cube and water instead of from meat and vegetables. If you do make your own, chill it quickly and lift off the fat when solid.

16. Always broil bacon, sausages, chops and beefburgers well —and on a rack. Surplus fat will drip off when cooking.

17. If you choose rice or pasta as the basis for a meal, then make lots of low fat sauce to keep the dish moist. Canned tomatoes are useful for sauces.

18. Choose moist fillings for sandwiches, such as cottage cheese, meat paste and tomatoes, bananas or canned fish and canned fish and lemon juice so you don't have to use butter or margarine as well.

19. In chicken dishes, if thighs or legs are substituted for breasts, the fat count will increase, since dark meat is fattier than white. Whichever is used, be sure to remove skin.

20. Ripe "homegrown" tomatoes can be substituted for canned tomatoes. However, only the juiciest, ripest tomatoes

should be used. If tomatoes are pink and hard and tasteless, canned tomatoes are much better.

21. Use spices, herbs and low fat sauces on vegetables instead of butter or margarine.

You Can't Get Fat Without Fats

Fats provide nearly half the calories that the average person eats in a day and often we hardly notice we're eating them! Because so little fat supplies so many calories, just a modest reduction in your intake can mean surprising weight loss. Here are 7 tips that add up to a stay slim formula.

1. *Always measure.* Measure out a modest butter or margarine *total* allowance for yourself each day. It's the one sure way to guarantee that you aren't inadvertently soaring over your correct daily calorie intake by adding a little bit here and a little bit there when spreading and cooking throughout the day. Special low calorie spreads can clearly be helpful.

Not only are butter and margarine among the highest calorie foods, they are also the source of the most easily "forgotten" calories.

"What did you have for breakfast?"

"Oh—just a slice of toast!"

No mention of the margarine or butter spread on the toast, which can very often supply you with as many calories as the bread itself. Or more.

2. *Read that package.* Pick your packs of frozen food by first

reading the "how to cook" instructions on the labels. Many main dishes from the frozen-food cabinets are very modest in calories, and most can be grilled or otherwise cooked without adding fat.

With such a wide choice available, it's pointless to pick the comparatively few items—particularly those in batter—which can only be fried.

3. *Stop buttering vegetables.* You'll soon get out of the habit! Instead, make the finishing touch chopped parsley, chives, etc.

4. *Forget about prefrying.* After you have prepared vegetables for casseroles, soups and stews, skip the traditional prefrying stage. You'll hardly notice any difference in the final flavor. In fact, this omission makes one of the most effortless of major calorie savings.

5. *Use a little less.* Use a little bit less next time you mash butter or margarine into the potatoes or add it to any other dish. With fats, just a little means a lot of calories—even tiny economies are worthwhile. And since fats tend to be used frequently in the kitchen, lots of little savings can have a major reducing effect on your total daily calorie intake.

6. *Eat more white fish.* Because white fish is so low in fat content, it is very low in calories compared with other proteins. Fish —unless you fry it, of course—can help to balance out your weekly calorie intake by providing some very low calorie meals.

7. *Think fats.* Consider the probable fat content every time you need to choose from an unfamiliar menu. All low fat meals are reasonably modest in calories; all high fat meals must be high. Fats are the *main* factor to consider in choosing weight-wise food.

A 7-Unit Low Fat Meal Plan

Here are suggested meals for a week to show you how easy it is to eat the 7-Unit Low Fat way: tasty, nourishing meals which will satisfy your hunger and peel off those unwanted pounds. We've even provided afternoon snacks.

Each meal is valued in fat units. Notice how crammed with treats each day's weight-wise menu is. And know that by the end of the day you will have consumed only 7 fat units!

SUNDAY

Breakfast

3 Ginger Muffins* or 1 cup raisin bran and 4 oz. skim milk
6 oz. apple juice
Coffee or tea

Total fat units = 1

Lunch

Vegetable Noodle Soup*
4 oz. low fat cottage cheese
1 tomato, cut in wedges

---

* Indicates recipe contained in book.

1 slice whole wheat bread
Coffee or tea

Total fat units = 3

Midafternoon snack

1 cup low fat yogurt with chopped fresh peach, pear or plum
Total fat units = ½

Dinner

Chicken Bavarian*
Baked Potato with Cheese Topping*
Chestnut Waldorf Salad*
Banana Whip*
Coffee or tea

Total fat units = 2½
Total fat units for the day: 7

MONDAY

Breakfast

2 Shredded Wheat biscuits (without sugar)
4 oz. skim milk
½ cup sliced peaches, fresh or canned waterpack, drained
Coffee or tea

Total fat units = 1

Lunch

Open-faced sandwich:
1 slice rye or pumpernickel bread
3½ oz. light meat chicken
Lettuce, tomato slices and mustard
Coffee or tea

Total fat units = 2

Midafternoon snack

Carrot and cucumber sticks and green pepper strips

* Indicates recipe contained in book.

Zesty Yogurt Dip*

Total fat units = 0

Dinner

Chili*
½ cup cooked white rice
Turnip Slaw* or Cole Slaw*
Plum Pudding* or canned waterpack plums
Coffee or tea

Total fat units = 4
Total fat units for the day: 7

TUESDAY

Breakfast

6 oz. orange juice
4 oz. low fat cottage cheese
1 bran muffin
Coffee or tea

Total fat units = 2

Lunch

Salad: 1 hard-boiled egg, sliced with sliced tomatoes,
    cucumbers, mushrooms, green onions, and greens
    mixed with 1 tablespoon Parmesan cheese and Tomato
    Salad Dressing*
Coffee or tea

Total fat units = 2½

Midafternoon snack

1 apple and 1 cup unbuttered popcorn

Total fat units = 0

Dinner

Mint Chicken Breasts*
Potato Salad*

---

* Indicates recipe contained in book.

1 cup green beans, cooked and sprinkled with chopped
     parsley
½ cantaloupe, with wedge of lemon or canned waterpack
     pear halves
Coffee or tea

Total fat units = 2½
Total fat units for the day: 7

WEDNESDAY

Breakfast

½ grapefruit
½ cup cooked oatmeal with cinnamon and 1 tablespoon
     raisins
4 oz. skim milk
Coffee or tea

Total fat units = 1

Lunch

Tuna Tortillas*
2 canned waterpack pear halves
Coffee or tea

Total fat units = 1½

Midafternoon snack

1 orange and 2 celery sticks

Total fat units = 0

Dinner

Veal Curry*
Tossed Salad: greens with sliced green peppers and chopped
     green onions, with Tomato Salad Dressing*
Apple Crunch*
Coffee or tea

Total fat units = 4½
Total fat units for the day: 7

---

* Indicates recipe contained in book.

THURSDAY

Breakfast

    6 oz. tomato juice
    1 poached egg
    1 slice whole wheat toast
    Coffee or tea

                        Total fat units = 2½

Lunch

    Chef Salad: crisp greens, cauliflower, celery, ½ oz. cheese
        (Monterey, Edam or Muenster)
    5 saltine crackers
    2 slices canned waterpack pineapple
    Coffee or tea

                        Total fat units = 1½

Midafternoon snack

    1 apple and 2 plums

                        Total fat units = 0

Dinner

    Chicken in a Pot*
    Salad of sliced tomatoes and onions, topped with Tomato
        Salad Dressing* and sprinkled with 1 teaspoon lemon
        juice
    Fruit and Rice*
    Coffee or tea

                        Total fat units = 3
                    Total fat units for the day: 7

FRIDAY

Breakfast

    1 orange, peeled and sliced into rounds, topped with ½ cup
        low fat plain yogurt, sprinkled with ½ teaspoon grated
        lemon rind

* Indicates recipe contained in book.

1 bran muffin
Coffee or tea

Total fat units $= 1\frac{1}{4}$

Lunch

1 glass tomato juice with celery stick swizzler
1 slice whole wheat bread, topped with ¼ cup Cottage
    Cheese Carrot Spread*
1 wedge cantaloupe with lemon
Coffee or tea

Total fat units $= 1\frac{1}{2}$

Midafternoon snack

1 cup unsweetened applesauce sprinkled with cinnamon

Total fat units $= 0$

Dinner

Split-Pea Soup*
Baked Fillets of Fish*
Steamed Spinach with Nutmeg*
½ cup cooked brown rice
Salad: sliced cucumbers with dill Tomato Salad Dressing*
Baked Bananas*
Coffee or tea

Total fat units $= 4\frac{1}{4}$
Total fat units for the day: 7

SATURDAY

Breakfast

1 medium navel orange
1 hard- or soft-boiled egg
Coffee or tea

Total fat units $= 2$

---

* Indicates recipe contained in book.

Lunch

Gazpacho* or vegetable soup
Macaroni Salad*
Coffee or tea

Total fat units = 1

Midafternoon snack

1 banana and 4 carrot sticks

Total fat units = 0

Dinner

Stuffed Mushrooms*
Paella*
Tossed Salad: greens, sliced red onion, sliced cucumbers
    with Tomato Salad Dressing*
2 slices Apple Oatmeal Loaf*
Coffee or tea

Total fat units = 4
Total fat units for the day: 7

* Indicates recipe contained in book.

111 7-Unit Low Fat Diet Recipes
(Each recipe serves 2)

Here are 111 recipes—easy to fix, delicious and nutritious—to help you peel off those unwanted pounds the 7-Unit Low Fat Diet way. You'll find recipes for every purpose from appetizers to desserts, prepared especially for you by a well-known American nutritionist.

We want to call your attention especially to the pasta section. Low fat dieting brings you the freedom to eat foods you enjoy at a calorie cost that will slim you—and puts carbohydrate food like pasta into a new, more realistic perspective. You can eat all the pasta you want, as long as you curb the real culprit on the plate—fat. Our recipes with innovative sauces show you how.

And don't miss four delicious ways to serve baked potatoes—zero fat units in themselves—*without butter or sour cream!* There's even a way to fix French fried potatoes without using oil or fat. (See page 103.)

Take advantage of the brand name convenience foods which can be used under the 7-Unit Low Fat plan. They are listed on pages 141–183 in Part III, The Fat Units Counter.

Bon appétit!

APPETIZERS

CAULIFLOWER DIP

(½ fat unit per recipe)

1 head cauliflower (with leaves and center stem removed)
5 tablespoons low fat plain yogurt
1 teaspoon capers
1 teaspoon lemon juice
⅓ cup minced onion
1 teaspoon dry hot mustard
3 cloves garlic, minced
2 tablespoons minced parsley
Salt and pepper to taste

Steam cauliflower until tender. Place in an electric blender with yogurt and purée until smooth. Place the purée in a bowl; add all other ingredients. Chill mixture for at least 1 hour. Serve with raw vegetables.

Makes about 2 cups.

CURRIED LENTIL DIP

(0 fat units per recipe)

1 cup well-cooked lentils
½ cup chopped green pepper
2 tablespoons chopped onion
1 teaspoon curry powder
1 tablespoon low fat plain yogurt
1 tablespoon canned tomato paste
Salt to taste

Place all ingredients in blender and purée until smooth. Chill for at least 2 hours. Serve with French bread or pita bread, which must be calculated separately.

Makes about 1½ cups.

DILLED SHRIMP WITH CELERY

(¾ fat unit per recipe)

4 ounces large shrimp
2 teaspoons low fat plain yogurt
2 tablespoons minced onion
2 teaspoons undiluted frozen unsweetened orange-juice
   concentrate
½ teaspoon dill weed
2 teaspoons lemon juice
Salt and pepper to taste
4 stalks celery

Drop shrimp into boiling water and cook until they turn pink, about 4 minutes. Remove from hot water, peel, and chop fine. Add all other ingredients (except celery) and mix well. Clean celery and cut into pieces about 3 inches long. Fill with shrimp mixture and sprinkle with more dill weed. Chill, and serve as appetizers.

Makes about ¾ cup.

TANGY SCALLOP SEVICHE

(¾ fat unit per recipe)

4 ounces raw sea scallops
½ cup lemon juice
1 teaspoon dried red pepper
Black pepper to taste
1 tablespoon chopped onion
1 teaspoon minced celery
1 tablespoon minced fresh red pepper or canned pimiento
Salt to taste

Cut scallops into quarters. Add lemon juice, red pepper and black pepper. Marinate in refrigerator 6–8 hours. When ready to serve, drain off juice, add other ingredients, mix, and serve.

Serves 2.

STUFFED MUSHROOMS

(½ fat unit per recipe)

4 large mushrooms (or 8 small ones)
3 tablespoons low fat plain yogurt
2 tablespoons minced onion
1 tablespoon minced green pepper
2 tablespoons minced water chestnuts
1 tablespoon lemon juice
½ teaspoon curry powder

Clean mushrooms and remove stems and mince them. Combine remaining ingredients, plus minced mushroom stems. Stuff mushroom caps with mixture. Twist pepper grinder a few times over mushrooms. Sprinkle with additional lemon juice and place under broiler until hot and light brown.

Serves 4.

COTTAGE CHEESE CARROT SPREAD

(1 fat unit per recipe)

1 cup low fat cottage cheese
½ cup grated carrots
2 tablespoons chopped chives
1 teaspoon Worcestershire sauce

Combine all ingredients. Refrigerate in a tightly covered container until ready to use.

Serves 4 as a spread.

ZESTY YOGURT DIP

(1 fat unit per recipe)

1 cup low fat plain yogurt
4 green olives stuffed with pimiento, chopped
1 tablespoon grated onion
1 teaspoon white prepared horseradish
1 teaspoon Worcestershire sauce

Combine all ingredients. Refrigerate to allow flavors to blend. Use as a dip for crudités.

Makes about 1 cup.

SOUPS

MINESTRONE

(1 fat unit per serving)

2 cups canned peeled tomatoes, with juice
1 cup kidney beans (cooked)*
1½ cups chicken stock (see page 118)
1 cup chopped onions
½ cup chopped celery
1 tablespoon marjoram
1 clove garlic, minced
Black pepper and salt to taste
1 cup macaroni
½ cup uncooked green peas

Place all ingredients except macaroni and peas into a heavy pot. Bring to boil and simmer for 15 minutes. Add macaroni and peas, bring to boil; lower heat and simmer 8–10 minutes.

Serves 4.

BORSCHT

(½ fat unit per serving)

2½ cups diced beets
⅓ cup sliced carrots
¾ cup sliced onions
¾ cup canned tomatoes, with juice
⅓ cup chicken stock (see page 118)
3 tablespoons lemon juice
3 tablespoons vinegar
½ teaspoon dry horseradish
1½ teaspoons dill weed
Salt and pepper to taste

Cook beets, carrots and onions in a small amount of water until

* Canned kidney beans can be used; if so they should be drained.

tender. Combine all ingredients in electric blender or food processor and purée. Chill. If desired, top each serving with a dollop of low fat plain yogurt.

Serves 4.

NEW ORLEANS CHICKEN GUMBO

(3½ fat units per serving)

1 large chicken breast, skinned
2 ounces very lean pork
½ cup chicken stock (see page 118)
1½ cups canned tomatoes, with juice
1 cup chopped onions
¾ cup diced green pepper
2 large cloves garlic, chopped
4 tablespoons lemon juice
2 tablespoons arrowroot
1 tablespoon thyme
10 drops Tabasco
Salt and black pepper to taste
½ cup scallops or shrimp, raw
1 cup cut-up okra
2 teaspoons gumbo filé powder*

Poach the chicken, in water to cover, until meat is opaque and tender, about 20 minutes. Cool; strip chicken from bones and cut into small pieces. Set aside. Cut pork into bite-size pieces. Brown in a large heavy pot. Drain off fat. Add chicken stock, ½ cup of the tomatoes, onion, green pepper, garlic and lemon juice. Stir in arrowroot. Add thyme and Tabasco, season with salt and pepper, and simmer, covered, for 30 minutes, stirring from time to time.

Add chicken, scallops or shrimp, okra, and the remainder of tomatoes and juice. Bring to a boil and simmer, covered, for 15 minutes. Add gumbo filé powder and stir; do not boil. Serve over cooked brown rice.

Serves 2.

---

* Gumbo filé powder is made from sassafras leaves, and used in New Orleans cooking.

CRANBERRY SOUP

(½ fat unit per serving)

2 cups fresh cranberries
1 cup minced carrots
¼ cup chopped onions
1½ cups chicken stock (see page 118)
¼ cup canned peeled tomatoes, strained
2 tablespoons undiluted frozen unsweetened orange-juice
     concentrate
½ teaspoon dill weed

In heavy saucepan, simmer cranberries, carrots and onions in ½ cup water for about 15 minutes, or until all liquid is absorbed. Place all ingredients in blender. Purée. Chill. If desired, top each serving with one tablespoon low fat plain yogurt and sprinkle with minced chives or the green part of scallions.

Serves 2.

GAZPACHO

(½ fat unit per serving)

1¾ cups canned tomatoes, strained
¾ cup chicken stock (see page 118)
½ cup sliced green pepper
½ small onion, cut into rings
½ cup peeled and sliced cucumber
3 tablespoons vinegar
2 cloves garlic, minced
1 teaspoon basil
3 drops Tabasco
Salt and pepper to taste

Combine all ingredients in a large bowl and chill for at least 3 hours. Serve with ½ cup croutons (made from 1 ounce French bread and toasted in oven).

Serves 2.

VEGETABLE NOODLE SOUP

(2 fat units per serving)

3½ cups vegetable stock (see page 119)
½ cup minced onion
½ cup canned tomatoes, with juice
1 teaspoon thyme
1 teaspoon basil
1 cup cut-up vegetables. (Use any of the following vegetables: zucchini, mushrooms, green beans, peas, cauliflower, celery, carrots, corn. The more variety, the better the soup.)
¾ cup spinach noodles
A few cabbage leaves, shredded
Salt and pepper to taste

Place chicken stock, onions, tomatoes, thyme and basil in a heavy saucepan and bring to a boil. Lower heat; add cup-up vegetables and simmer for 10 minutes. Add noodles, shredded cabbage, salt and pepper; simmer until noodles are al dente.

Serves 4.

TURKEY RICE SOUP

(1 fat unit per serving)

4 cups turkey stock (see page 118)
⅓ cup brown rice
2 tablespoons minced onion
2 teaspoons marjoram
1 cup green beans, cut into small pieces
½ cup peas
Salt and pepper to taste

Place stock in a heavy saucepan; add rice, onion and marjoram. Bring to a boil, lower heat and simmer, covered, for 30 minutes. Add beans and peas, salt and pepper to taste; simmer for another 10–15 minutes. If soup needs thinning, add up to 1 cup additional stock, and heat through. Add 1 fat unit for each additional cup of turkey stock.

Serves 4.

BLENDER ASPARAGUS SOUP

(1 fat unit per serving)

4 cups chopped asparagus* (fresh, canned or frozen)
3 cups skim milk
3 tablespoons chopped onions
3 tablespoons lemon juice
1 tablespoon tarragon
Salt and pepper to taste

Set aside half the chopped asparagus. Place all other ingredients in a heavy saucepan, bring to a boil; lower heat and simmer for 20 minutes. Cool 10–15 minutes. Place mixture in electric blender or food processor and purée. Return mixture to saucepan, bring to a boil, and add the remaining 2 cups asparagus. Lower heat and simmer for 10 minutes. If desired, top with paper-thin lemon slices, or a dollop of low fat plain yogurt before serving.

Serves 4.

SPLIT-PEA SOUP

(2¼ fat units per serving)

2 ounces pork sausage links
2 cups yellow split peas, soaked and drained
1 cup chopped onions
¼ cup chopped celery
¾ cup canned tomatoes, with juice
1 cup chicken stock (see page 118)
1 teaspoon rosemary

Cut sausage links into ½-inch pieces. Bake in a 350° F. oven 10–15 minutes, or until brown. Drain on paper towels. Place in a heavy saucepan, add all other ingredients. Cover with water, bring to a boil, then lower heat and simmer for 2½ hours, stirring from time to time.

Makes 4 servings.

---

* Broccoli, beans or peas may be substituted for asparagus.

LENTIL SOUP

(0 fat units per serving)

2 cups well-cooked lentils
1 small onion (cooked with lentils)
1½ cups canned tomatoes, with juice
1 garlic clove, minced
2 tablespoons minced parsley
1 teaspoon lemon juice
½ cup minced celery
1 tablespoon basil
5 drops Tabasco

Purée lentils and onion in electric blender. Add tomatoes and blend again. Put in a saucepan, and add all other ingredients. Bring to a boil; lower heat, and simmer for 15 minutes. Add black pepper and salt to taste before serving.

Serves 4.

PUMPKIN SOUP

(½ fat unit per serving)

2 cups puréed pumpkin, fresh or canned
1 cup clam or mussel broth
½ cup skim milk
¼ cup minced onion
¼ teaspoon ground cloves
¼ teaspoon cayenne pepper

Mix pumpkin and clam broth with wire whisk until smooth. Place in saucepan and bring to boil. Lower heat; add other ingredients, and simmer for 10 minutes.

Serves 4.

BEAN AND BARLEY SOUP

(½ fat unit per serving)

4 cups vegetable stock (see page 119)
⅓ cup barley
½ cup chopped onions
1½ cups sliced mushrooms and/or green beans, cut into
    ½-inch pieces

1 teaspoon oregano
1 tablespoon minced parsley
Black pepper and salt to taste

Bring stock to boil in heavy pot. Add barley and onions, lower heat, and simmer for 45 minutes. Add rest of vegetables and seasonings and simmer 15–20 minutes longer.

Serves 4.

FISH

TUNA SALAD

(1½ fat units per serving)

2½ cups alfalfa sprouts or shredded lettuce
5 tablespoons chopped green onions
1 cup sliced mushrooms
6 tablespoons Tomato Salad Dressing (see page 119)
1 7-ounce can solid white tuna, waterpack, drained, and broken
    into small chunks
½ cup peeled and sliced cucumber
1 teaspoon dill weed
½ cup low fat plain yogurt
2 tablespoons minced parsley

Place 2 cups alfalfa sprouts or lettuce in a glass bowl; sprinkle with 2 tablespoons chopped green onions. Top with mushrooms. Add Tomato Salad Dressing, tuna, and the rest of the green onions.

Combine the cucumber, dill and yogurt; spoon over salad, and top with the rest of the alfalfa sprouts or lettuce and the parsley. Chill well before serving.

Serves 4.

TUNA TORTILLAS

(1½ fat units per serving)

4 corn tortillas
1 cup shredded lettuce or alfalfa sprouts

FILLING:

1 7-ounce can solid white tuna (waterpacked), drained and
    flaked
2 teaspoons undiluted frozen unsweetened orange-juice
    concentrate
¼ cup minced celery
⅓ cup low fat plain yogurt
½ cup minced green onion
2 hard-boiled eggs (whites only), chopped
1 tablespoon lemon juice
1 teaspoon Dijon mustard
1 teaspoon dry hot mustard
Black pepper and salt to taste

Combine all filling ingredients. Fold each tortilla in half, and place all four in a pan just big enough to hold them. Fill each tortilla with tuna mixture. Bake in a 350° F. oven for 15 minutes. Remove from oven; top with lettuce or sprouts, and serve.

Serves 4.

FISH CHOWDER

(1 fat unit per serving)

8 ounces salt cod, or other low fat fish
1 ounce lean pork, finely diced
1½ cups peeled and diced potatoes
¾ cup diced celery
3 cups canned tomatoes, with juice
¾ cup clam juice or broth, or fish broth
1½ cups diced onions
¼ cup diced green pepper
1 tablespoon thyme
Pepper to taste

Soak cod in cold water for 10 hours, or overnight, changing water several times. Drain, and cut into small pieces. Combine all ingredients, except the fish, in a heavy pot. Bring to boil, lower heat, and simmer for about 20 minutes. Add fish, bring to a boil, lower heat, and simmer until fish flakes, about 10–15 minutes.

Serves 4.

PAELLA

(2½ fat units per serving)

½ cup chopped onions
½ cup minced green pepper
3 cloves garlic, minced
½ cup long grain brown rice, raw
1½ cups canned tomatoes, with juice
¼ teaspoon saffron powder
½ teaspoon oregano
¾ cup chicken stock (see page 118)
1 ounce hot link sausages, cut into ½-inch pieces
½ large chicken breast, skinned and boned (about 3½ ounces), slivered
2 ounces scallops (quartered, if large)
½ cup green peas, fresh or frozen
1 tablespoon fresh red pepper, or pimiento, chopped
Pepper and salt to taste
2 clams

Sauté onions, green pepper and garlic in a nonstick frying pan. Add rice, stir, and add tomatoes, saffron, oregano and ½ cup chicken stock. Simmer gently for 35 minutes. In separate nonstick pan, brown sausage. Drain off fat. Add sausage to rice mixture, and add chicken, scallops, peas, red pepper or pimiento and the rest of the chicken stock. Add salt and pepper to taste.

Place mixture in a casserole, cover and bake in a 350° F. oven until rice is done (about 20 minutes). About four minutes before casserole has finished cooking, remove lid, place 2 clams on top and put back in oven until clams have opened.

Serves 2.

OLD-FASHIONED SALMON LOAF

(3½ fat units per serving)

1 egg, plus white of one egg
7¾-ounce can salmon, drained, cleaned and flaked
¼ cup low fat plain yogurt
¼ cup minced onion
2 tablespoons minced celery
½ teaspoon fennel seed
½ teaspoon dill seed
¼ cup sliced mushrooms
¼ cup tiny pieces of corn tortilla, untoasted
Black pepper and salt to taste
Paprika

Beat egg and egg white until thick and yellow. Combine all other ingredients in a bowl; then fold eggs into mixture. Place mixture into two individual ramekins, or one small casserole. Sprinkle with paprika. Bake in oven for 35 minutes at 350° F. Serve with Fish Sauce (see page 118).

Serves 2.

BAKED FILLETS OF FISH

(1½ fat units per serving)

1 large cucumber
8 ounces striped bass fillets (sole, cod, halibut or any other ½ unit fish listed in Fat Units Counter, page 134, may be used)
Black pepper to taste
Lemon juice
½ cup French bread cubes
1½ tablespoons minced parsley
1½ teaspoons tarragon
1 teaspoon capers
¼ cup minced onion
½ lemon
4 tablespoons low fat plain yogurt

Peel cucumber and cut in half lengthwise. Scoop out all seeds. Cut lengthwise again so that there are four pieces. Cut these into ½-inch pieces. Sprinkle flesh side of fish fillets with black pepper and lemon juice. Combine bread cubes, 1 teaspoon parsley, 1 teaspoon tarragon and the capers, and spoon mixture over flesh side of fillets. Gently roll each fillet so that skin is on outside. Secure with small metal picks or toothpicks and place in a shallow baking dish. Place cucumber pieces around the fish and sprinkle the onion and the rest of the parsley and tarragon over it. Squeeze a lemon half over all, and spoon the yogurt over the top. Bake uncovered in a 400° F. oven for 15 minutes. Lower heat to 350° F. and continue baking for an additional 30 minutes.

Serves 2.

POACHED FISH FILLETS

(1 fat unit per serving)

12 ounces fillet of flounder
1 cup water
2 tablespoons lemon juice
1 tablespoon grated onion
1 tablespoon dill weed
Salt and pepper to taste

Arrange fillets in a large skillet. Add water and lemon juice. Sprinkle fillets with onion, dill weed, and salt and pepper. Cover and simmer 6–8 minutes, or until fish flakes easily. Remove fish with a slotted pancake turner. Serve at once.

Serves 2.

BAKED SWORDFISH WITH ORANGE

(2½ fat units per serving)

8 ounces swordfish steak, cut into small chunks
¾ cup canned tomatoes, with juice
½ cup minced celery
3 tablespoons minced onion
2 tablespoons undiluted frozen unsweetened orange-juice
    concentrate
½ teaspoon ground celery seed
½ teaspoon fennel seed
Salt and pepper to taste

Place fish in shallow baking dish. Combine all other ingredients; pour over fish, and bake in 350° F. oven for about 30 minutes.

Serves 2.

POULTRY

MINT CHICKEN BREASTS

(2 fat units per serving)

1 large chicken breast, skinned, split in half
¼ cup lemon juice
¼ cup chicken stock (see page 118)
1 small onion, chopped
1 teaspoon dried mint
Salt and pepper to taste
2 cups alfalfa sprouts

Place chicken in a nonstick skillet over low heat. Add lemon juice, chicken stock, onion, mint, salt and pepper. Simmer, covered, for about 20 to 25 minutes. Add alfalfa sprouts and simmer for 5 minutes more, or until sprouts are hot and slightly wilted.

Serves 2.

CHICKEN AND SHRIMP CREOLE

(3 fat units per serving)

1 ounce lean pork, cut into small pieces
½ large chicken breast, skinned, cut in strips
2½ cups canned tomatoes, with juice
½ cup brown rice, raw
1 cup chopped green onion tops
¾ cup chicken stock (see page 118)
½ cup chopped green pepper
2 large cloves garlic, chopped
1 tablespoon thyme
Salt and black pepper to taste
10 large shrimp, peeled

Brown the pork in a large nonstick skillet; drain off any fat that accumulates. Add all other ingredients, except shrimp. Bring to a boil; lower heat and simmer 50–60 minutes with lid on. Add shrimp and cook for another 4–5 minutes, until shrimp turn pink.

Serves 2.

COUNTRY CHICKEN

(3 fat units per serving)

1½ cups sliced mushrooms
¾ cup chopped onion
3 cloves garlic, minced
½ large green pepper, sliced
1 cup sliced okra
¾ cup barley
1½ cups chicken stock (see page 118)
10 drops Tabasco
1 tablespoon oregano
½ teaspoon ground celery seed
Black pepper and salt to taste
1 large chicken breast, skinned, split in half

In a nonstick frying pan, sauté mushrooms, onion, garlic, green pepper and okra 8–10 minutes, stirring constantly. Remove from heat and add barley, stirring well. Place mixture in a deep casserole dish. Add chicken stock and seasonings. Top with chicken breast halves, flesh side down. Bake covered in a 325° F. oven 60–70 minutes, or until all liquid has been absorbed.

Serves 2.

CHICKEN AND BULGUR WHEAT

(3½ fat units per serving)

1 whole chicken breast, skinned
1 cup chicken stock (see page 118)
½ cup bulgur wheat
1 egg, beaten
1 teaspoon dry hot mustard
2 teaspoons Dijon mustard
1 cup peeled and chopped cucumbers
1 ripe tomato, chopped
1 cup chopped green onions, including tops
1 teaspoon dill weed
10 drops Tabasco
Salt and pepper to taste

(Continued)

Poach chicken breast in water for 20 minutes. Cool, strip meat from bones, and cut meat into slivers. Set aside. Bring chicken stock to a boil in a heavy saucepan; lower heat, add bulgur wheat, and stir over low heat until all liquid has been absorbed. Remove from heat; stir in slightly beaten egg and both mustards. Add all remaining ingredients; mix well, cool and then chill. Serve on salad greens.

Serves 2.

SWEET AND SOUR CHICKEN

(1½ fat units per serving)

    1 large chicken breast, skinned
    2 cups shredded cabbage
    ¼ cup minced white onion
    Salt and pepper to taste
    1 small orange, peeled and divided into segments

SWEET AND SOUR SAUCE:
    ½ cup undiluted frozen unsweetened apple-juice concentrate
    2 tablespoons vinegar
    1 teaspoon dry horseradish
    Dash of cayenne pepper

Poach chicken breast in water. Cool, and cut into strips. Place cabbage in the bottom of a casserole; add chicken, and sprinkle with onion. Add salt and pepper. Arrange orange segments over the top. Combine all sauce ingredients; pour sauce over all. Bake in a 350° F. oven for 40 minutes.

Serves 2.

CHICKEN BAVARIAN

(2 fat units per serving)

    2 cups cooked lentils
    4 large cloves garlic, minced
    12 thin raw onion rings
    Salt and pepper to taste
    1 large chicken breast, skinned, split in half
    2 cups sauerkraut, with a little juice
    5 crushed juniper berries
    1 cup canned tomatoes, with juice

Place cooked lentils in the bottom of a baking dish or nonstick pan. Add half the garlic, onion rings, salt and pepper. Add the two halves of chicken breast and the rest of the garlic. Cover the mixture with half the sauerkraut and juice; sprinkle with juniper berries. Top with the rest of the sauerkraut and then a layer of tomatoes. Bake, uncovered, in a 350° F. oven for 50 minutes.

Serves 2.

CHICKEN IN A POT

(2 fat units per serving)

2 chicken breast halves, skinned, bone intact
2 medium onions, peeled
2 turnips, peeled
4 carrots, scraped, cut in half
2 big wedges of cabbage
2 small potatoes, peeled
6 cloves garlic, peeled
1 quart water

MUSTARD SAUCE:
½ cup low fat plain yogurt
1 teaspoon Dijon mustard
Salt and pepper to taste

Place all ingredients (except Mustard Sauce) in a heavy saucepan. Bring to a boil. Lower heat; cover, and simmer 45–50 minutes. Combine Mustard Sauce ingredients; add to chicken mixture, and serve very hot.

Serves 2.

COLD CHICKEN AND FRUIT

(3 fat units per serving)

1½ chicken breasts, skinned and boned
1 cup seedless grapes
¼ cup minced green pepper
1 cup chopped nectarines or peeled peaches
½ cup sliced plums
4 tablespoons minced red Bermuda onion (optional)
Pepper to taste

(Continued)

ORANGE DRESSING:
>   1 cup chicken stock (see page 118)
>   ⅓ cup undiluted frozen unsweetened orange-juice concentrate
>   1 teaspoon rosemary
>   2 teaspoons arrowroot
>   Pepper to taste

Poach chicken breasts in water. Strip the meat from the bones and cut into slivers. Place in a bowl with grapes (cut in half), green pepper, nectarines or peaches, and plums. Add red onion, if desired. Add pepper.

In a saucepan, combine chicken stock, orange juice, rosemary, arrowroot and pepper. Beat with a wire whisk. Bring to a boil, then immediately lower heat and simmer, stirring constantly, until sauce is thickened. Chill.

Mix salad and dressing. Garnish with additional rosemary and pepper. Chill.

Serves 2.

CHICKEN IN RAMEKINS

(1½ fat units per serving)

>   1 large uncooked chicken breast, skinned
>   1 clove garlic, minced
>   1½ cups sliced mushrooms
>   1 cup minced onion
>   ¼ cup undiluted frozen unsweetened orange-juice concentrate
>   3 tablespoons water

Strip meat from chicken breast and slice into small pieces. Place half the chicken in the bottom of individual ramekins. Cover with garlic and mushrooms, top with the rest of the chicken and spread the onion over the top. Mix the orange juice and water; pour over each ramekin. Bake uncovered in a 350° F. oven for 1 hour.

Serves 2.

CREAMED CHICKEN

(3 fat units per serving)

>   3 chicken breast halves, skinned
>   1 cup green peas
>   1 cup sliced mushrooms
>   ½ cup sliced green onion tops

1 tablespoon thyme
1 tablespoon lemon juice
2 tablespoons dry hot mustard
Salt and pepper to taste

CREAM SAUCE:
    2 cups skim milk
    1 tablespoon arrowroot
    2 tablespoons chicken stock (see page 118)
    Salt and pepper to taste

Poach chicken breast halves for 20 minutes. Cool, remove meat, and cut into small strips.

Stir Cream Sauce ingredients over low heat, with a wire whisk, until sauce thickens, about 15 minutes. Add chicken and all other ingredients; simmer for about 15 minutes, and serve over cooked rice, noodles or potatoes.

Serves 2.

CHICKEN DIVAN PUFF

(3 fat units per serving)

1 large chicken breast, skinned
2 cups asparagus, chopped into small pieces
½ lemon
1 whole egg
3 egg whites
Black pepper to taste
½ cup low fat plain yogurt
1 tablespoon vinegar
1 teaspoon thyme

Poach chicken breast in water to cover, until meat is opaque and partially cooked, about 15–20 minutes. Strip meat from breast, cut into small pieces, and place in the bottom of one casserole or two individual ramekins. Steam asparagus until tender, 10–15 minutes. Place on top of chicken; squeeze lemon juice over all.

Beat egg and egg whites together with a wire whisk, until foamy. Add black pepper to taste.

Combine yogurt, vinegar and thyme; beat into egg mixture. Pour mixture over chicken and asparagus. Bake uncovered in a 350° F. oven for 50 minutes.

Serves 2.

CHICKEN FLORENTINE

(2 fat units per serving)

½ large chicken breast, skinned
6 egg whites
1 teaspoon dry hot mustard
1 teaspoon minced onion
1 cup chicken stock (see page 118)
1 cup tightly packed chopped frozen, thawed, or fresh spinach
1½ cups cubed French bread
½ cup sliced mushrooms
½ teaspoon nutmeg
½ teaspoon celery seed
½ teaspoon sage
Black pepper and salt to taste

Poach chicken in water for 20 minutes; strip meat from bones and cut into small slivers. Beat egg whites, mustard and onion together with electric mixer until thick and pale yellow. Add chicken stock; beat well. Add all remaining ingredients to egg mixture. Pour batter into a casserole and bake in a 325° F. oven for 1 hour.

Serves 2.

BAKED CHICKEN ORIENTAL

(2 fat units per serving)

1 whole chicken breast, skinned
1 cup chopped onions
2 cloves garlic, minced
½ medium-size green pepper, slivered
¼ cup minced shallots
1 cup sliced mushrooms
2 medium baking potatoes, peeled and sliced
1 cup chicken stock (see page 118)
¼ cup sliced water chestnuts
1 tablespoon thyme
1 tablespoon soy sauce
Black pepper and salt to taste

Simmer chicken breast in a small amount of water for about 20 minutes, or until opaque; remove bones and cut chicken meat into slivers. Place in a Dutch oven with remaining ingredients. Bake in a 350° F. oven for 1 hour.

Serves 2.

STUFFED CORNISH GAME HENS

(3 fat units per hen)

2 fresh Cornish game hens, about 20 ounces each
½ cup vinegar or apple juice, for basting

STUFFING:

1 egg white, slightly beaten
½ cup fresh cranberries, rinsed and drained
1 tangerine, peeled, seeded, segments cut in half
¼ teaspoon mace
½ teaspoon ground coriander
Black pepper to taste
3 tablespoons minced celery

Wash and dry hens. Mix all stuffing ingredients together; stuff hens and skewer openings shut. Tie legs together. Roast hens in a 350° F. oven, breast side down, 40–45 minutes. Baste occasionally with vinegar or apple juice. Turn hens breast side up and continue baking for 15 minutes more.

Serves 2.

MEAT

LAMB STEW

(3 fat units per serving)

6 ounces lean lamb meat, cut from leg, cut into bite-size pieces
2½ cups water
1½ cups peeled and cut potato, large chunks
1 turnip, peeled and cut into large chunks
3 carrots, scraped and cut in half
1 cup sliced onions
½ cup diced celery
¼ cup barley
3 cloves garlic, minced
2 tablespoons minced parsley
1 teaspoon curry powder
½ teaspoon ground celery seed
½ teaspoon marjoram
Black pepper and salt to taste
1 cup green beans
½ cup green peas

Brown meat in a heavy pot. Drain off any fat that accumulates.
Add all other ingredients (except beans and peas), bring to boil,
lower heat, and simmer for 35 minutes. Add beans and peas and
simmer for 15 minutes longer.

Serves 2.

MEATBALLS ST. GERMAIN

(3½ fat units per serving)

MEATBALLS:

6 ounces lean ground beef
2 tablespoons low fat cottage cheese
1½ tablespoons fine plain bread crumbs
1 egg white, slightly beaten
2 tablespoons minced onion
Salt and black pepper to taste

Combine all ingredients; shape into 12 small balls. Brown in a nonstick skillet; drain off fat and set aside.

SAUCE:

¾ cup chopped onions
¼ cup chopped green onion tops
2 cloves garlic, chopped
¼ cup chopped green pepper
1 cup cooked green split peas, drained
1½ cups thinly sliced and peeled baking potatoes
Salt and pepper to taste
1 cup canned tomatoes, with juice

In a nonstick skillet, sauté both kinds of onion, garlic and green pepper until soft, about 5 minutes. Place peas in the bottom of a casserole; add potatoes and sprinkle with salt and pepper. Add meatballs, cooked vegetables, and pour tomatoes over all. Bake in a 350° F. oven for 1 hour.

Serves 2.

LIMA BEANS WITH BEEF

(4 fat units per serving)

6 ounces lean ground beef
1 cup chopped onions
3 tablespoons chopped green pepper
4 cloves garlic, chopped
2 cups lima beans, soaked for at least 3 hours and then drained, or frozen lima beans, thawed
6 tablespoons low fat cottage cheese
2½ cups canned tomatoes, with juice
½ cup corn, fresh, canned or frozen
1 tablespoon basil
1 teaspoon marjoram
Salt and black pepper to taste

Sauté beef in a nonstick skillet. Drain off any fat that accumulates. Add onion, green pepper and garlic; sauté 5–10 minutes, until vegetables are soft. Remove from heat. Add soaked lima beans. Add remaining ingredients, place in a casserole, and bake, uncovered, in a 350° F. oven for 1 hour. If frozen lima beans are used, bake for 20–30 minutes, until casserole is heated through.

Serves 2.

MEAT LOAF

(4 fat units per serving)

6 ounces lean ground beef
1 cup chopped onions
½ cup diced whole wheat bread
6 tablespoons low fat cottage cheese
2 cloves garlic, minced
1 teaspoon lemon juice
2 egg whites, slightly beaten
¼ cup chopped green pepper
1 teaspoon cayenne pepper
½ teaspoon dry hot mustard
Black pepper and salt to taste

Combine all ingredients. Bake, in a casserole dish or individual ramekins, for 1 hour in a 350° F. oven.

Serves 2.

CHILI

(3½ fat units per serving)

6 ounces ground round steak or chuck, crumbled
½ cup chopped green pepper
1¼ cups chopped onions
4 cloves garlic, minced
½ cup chopped celery
3 cups canned tomatoes, with juice
2 tablespoons chili powder
½ teaspoon ground cumin seed
1 teaspoon basil
1 teaspoon oregano
½ teaspoon ground coriander
½ teaspoon crushed dried red pepper
Black pepper to taste
1 cup cooked kidney beans
½ cup sliced mushrooms

Brown meat in heavy-bottomed pan. Stir to keep from sticking. If any fat accumulates, drain off. Add chopped pepper and onion, garlic and celery. Cook for about 5 minutes, stirring occasionally.

Add remaining ingredients except mushrooms and beans and bring to boil. Cover, lower heat and simmer at lowest heat for a minimum of 1 hour, stirring occasionally. Longer cooking makes a richer, more flavorful chili.

About 20 minutes before chili is ready, add mushrooms and kidney beans; stir well.

Serves 2.

STUFFED CABBAGE

(3½ fat units per serving)

1 small head cabbage
6 ounces lean ground beef
¾ cup chopped onions
1 cup sliced mushrooms
1 teaspoon tarragon
1 teaspoon lemon juice
Salt and black pepper to taste
1½ cups canned tomatoes, with juice
½ cup low fat plain yogurt
4 tablespoons undiluted frozen unsweetened orange-juice
    concentrate
1 teaspoon ground coriander

Gently cut away 6 large cabbage leaves from head. Parboil cabbage leaves until soft and flexible. Drain and set aside. Sauté beef in a nonstick frying pan until brown. Drain off any fat that accumulates. Add onions, mushrooms, tarragon, lemon juice, salt and pepper. Divide meat mixture among the cabbage leaves. Roll each leaf, with meat filling, into a little bundle, securing with a toothpick, if you desire. Place them, seam sides down, in a small casserole.

Combine tomatoes, yogurt, orange-juice concentrate and coriander and stir briskly with wire whisk. Pour over cabbage rolls. Bake in 350° F. oven for 45 minutes.

Serves 2.

BEEF, RICE AND BLACK BEAN CASSEROLE

(3½ fat units per serving)

½ cup raw brown rice
2 cups cooked black turtle beans
1 cup chicken stock (see page 118)
Salt and pepper to taste
4 ounces lean ground beef
½ cup chopped celery
¼ cup chopped green pepper
1 cup chopped onions
1 tablespoon minced mushrooms
1 tablespoon dried cilantro (coriander leaves)
2 cloves garlic, minced
1 teaspoon oregano

Place rice and 1 cup of water in a saucepan. Bring to a boil; lower heat, cover, and simmer 30–40 minutes, or until all water has been absorbed. Place beans in the bottom of a casserole dish and add rice. Pour chicken stock over mixture. Add salt and pepper.

Brown meat in a nonstick skillet. Drain off fat. Add vegetables and seasonings, and cook until vegetables are soft; stir mixture into rice-bean mixture. Bake in a 350° F. oven for 30 minutes.

Serves 2.

VEAL CURRY

(3½ fat units per serving)

4 ounces veal, ground or in small chunks
2 cups chopped onions
¾ cup chopped carrots
¾ cup chopped celery
1¼ cups diced raw potatoes
1 medium tart apple, unpeeled, diced
1 tablespoon curry powder
1 teaspoon lemon juice
1¼ cups chicken stock (see page 118)
¼ cup low fat plain yogurt

Brown the veal in a heavy pot. Drain off any fat that accumulates. Add onions, carrots, celery, potato and apple. Sprinkle with curry powder and lemon juice. Add ¾ cup of the chicken stock. Simmer, covered, for 2 hours. Halfway through, add the remaining ½ cup of chicken stock and the yogurt, mixing well.

Serve over 1½ cups cooked brown rice with these side dishes:
    ½ cup chopped green onion tops
    ½ cup minced green pepper
    ½ cup chopped water chestnuts
    1 pear, peeled, diced, and sprinkled with lemon juice

Serves 2.

VEAL WITH PINTO BEANS

(3½ fat units per serving)

    4 ounces lean veal, diced
    2 cups pinto beans, soaked and drained
    1½ cups diced onions
    ¾ cup diced carrots
    4 tablespoons undiluted frozen unsweetened orange-juice
        concentrate
    1¼ cups chicken stock (see page 118)
    3 cloves garlic, minced
    1 tablespoon dry hot mustard
    1 teaspoon whole celery seed

Brown veal in a nonstick frying pan. Drain off fat that may accumulate. Combine veal and remaining ingredients in a small pottery bean pot, or small casserole with tight-fitting lid. Cover and bake 4 hours in a 350° F. oven. Remove cover the last half-hour of baking, adding additional chicken stock if needed.

Serves 2.

PORK WITH CHICK PEAS

(2½ fat units per serving)

3 ounces lean pork, diced
½ cup canned chick peas, drained
2 cups diced squash (yellow or zucchini)
1 17-ounce can tomatoes, with juice
½ cup wheat pilaf (bulgur wheat)
2 tablespoons minced parsley
¼ cup minced onion
2 cloves garlic, minced
1 tablespoon cilantro (coriander leaves)
1 teaspoon oregano
2 tablespoons slivered raw red pepper or pimiento
Black pepper to taste

Brown pork in a nonstick frying pan; drain off fat. Combine all ingredients in a casserole; bake, uncovered, in a 350° F. oven 50–60 minutes.

Serves 2.

PORK HAWAIIAN

(4¾ fat units per serving)

6 ounces pork, fat removed, diced
½ cup unsweetened pineapple chunks
½ cup chopped orange segments
2 tablespoons sliced raw red pepper or pimiento
1 teaspoon soy sauce
½ cup minced onion
1 tablespoon vinegar
2 tablespoons low fat plain yogurt
¼ cup raw brown rice
3 tablespoons undiluted frozen unsweetened orange-juice
     concentrate
3 tablespoons water
Black pepper and salt to taste

Brown meat in a nonstick skillet. Drain off any fat that accumulates. Add rest of ingredients and bake in a small casserole, covered, in 350° F. oven for 1 hour.

Serves 2.

PASTAS

MACARONI AND CHEESE

(1½ fat units per serving)

2½ cups macaroni
1 cup low fat cottage cheese
1 teaspoon turmeric
Black pepper and salt to taste
1 cup chopped onions
¾ cup chopped green onion tops

SAUCE:

1 cup low fat milk
½ cup chicken stock (see page 118)
2 teaspoons arrowroot

Partially boil macaroni, drain, and place in the bottom of a casserole dish. Add cottage cheese, turmeric, and salt and pepper. Sauté onions and green onion tops in a nonstick frying pan. Add to macaroni mixture.

To make sauce, combine all ingredients in saucepan. Stir constantly, over low heat, with wire whisk, until sauce has thickened. Add sauce to casserole, and bake in 350° F. oven for 30 minutes.

Serves 2.

MACARONI SALAD

(½ fat unit per serving)

1½ cups cooked (al dente) macaroni, preferably whole wheat.
(Use elbow, seashell, or some other small pasta; a large,
denser pasta will not work with this recipe.)
½ cup cooked green peas
¼ cup low fat plain yogurt
1 tablespoon chili powder
½ cup minced green onion, including tops
¼ teaspoon ground cumin seed
Black pepper and salt to taste
¼ cup Tomato Salad Dressing (see page 119)
1 tablespoon chopped parsley

Combine all ingredients except Tomato Salad Dressing and parsley; chill. Just before serving, add dressing and sprinkle with parsley.

Serves 2.

FETTUCINE SALAD

(0 fat units per serving)

½ cup chopped broccoli
¾ cup chopped green onions, including tops
1½ cups sliced mushrooms
½ large green pepper, cut into thin slices
2 cloves garlic, minced
1 teaspoon grated lemon peel
1½ teaspoons basil
8 ounces fettucine
¾ cup Tomato Salad Dressing (see page 119)
¼ cup vinegar
1 teaspoon dry horseradish
4 drops Tabasco
Black pepper and salt to taste

Sauté the vegetables, garlic, lemon peel and basil in a nonstick frying pan, adding a little water; cook until tender but not soft. Set aside.

Cook fettucine in boiling salted water until it is al dente.

Meanwhile, combine Tomato Salad Dressing, vinegar, horse-radish and Tabasco into a sauce. Drain fettucine; toss with the sauce. Add cooked vegetables, pepper and salt. Serve at room temperature or chill.

Serves 2.

MACARONI AND BEEF CASSEROLE

(4 fat units per serving)

1½ cups macaroni (rotini, seashell or elbow)
1½ cups cooked navy beans
½ teaspoon cayenne pepper
8 ounces lean ground beef
¾ cup chopped onions
½ cup chopped celery
¼ cup chopped green pepper
2 tablespoons grated carrot
1 tablespoon lemon juice
2 cloves garlic, chopped
1 tablespoon basil
Black pepper and salt to taste
1¼ cups canned tomatoes, with juice
1 teaspoon capers

Partially cook macaroni in boiling water 3–5 minutes. Drain and put into casserole or nonstick pan. Place beans on top of macaroni and sprinkle with cayenne pepper. Brown the meat in a nonstick frying pan. Drain off all fat; add onion, celery, green pepper and carrot. Then add lemon juice, garlic, basil, salt and pepper. Cook until vegetables are soft and opaque. Add tomatoes and capers, and cook for 10 minutes longer, stirring occasionally. Pour over bean and macaroni mixture and bake, covered, in a 350° F. oven for 25 minutes.

Serves 2.

LASAGNE

(2½ fat units per serving)

4 ounces lean ground beef
1 17-ounce can tomatoes, with juice
⅔ cup chopped onions
½ cup sliced mushrooms
⅓ cup chopped green pepper
2 cloves garlic, minced
¼ cup chicken stock (see page 118)
2 tablespoons minced parsley
1½ teaspoons oregano
¼ teaspoon ground cloves
1 teaspoon basil
2 teaspoons lemon juice
Black pepper and salt to taste
4 ounces lasagna noodles
1 cup low fat cottage cheese

Brown meat in a nonstick skillet, and drain off any fat that accumulates. Add vegetables, seasonings, and chicken stock; bring to boil, lower heat, and simmer for 15 minutes.*

Cook lasagne noodles at high boil for 10 minutes. Do not overcook. Drain, run cold and then warm water over them. In a small, nonstick casserole, place a layer of sauce and then ¼ cup cottage cheese. Top with layer of half the noodles, then half the remaining sauce. Top sauce with remaining noodles, then remaining cottage cheese, cover with remaining sauce. Bake in a 350° F. oven, uncovered, 40–45 minutes. Let stand about 15 minutes before serving.

Serves 2.

SEASHELLS WITH CHICKEN AND BROCCOLI

(2 fat units per serving)

2 cups seashell macaroni
Black pepper and salt
1⅔ cups partially cooked chopped broccoli
1 large chicken breast, split in half, skinned

---

* Simmer same sauce for 25 minutes for use over spaghetti. Sauce with beef has 4¼ fat units per recipe, without beef ¼ fat unit.

SAUCE:

    ½ cup tarragon vinegar
    1½ cups canned tomatoes, with juice
    ¼ cup chopped onions
    ½ cup low fat plain yogurt
    ¼ cup sliced mushrooms
    1 teaspoon chili powder
    Black pepper and salt to taste

Parboil the macaroni, drain, and place in small casserole or a nonstick pan. Sprinkle with pepper and salt. Add broccoli, and place chicken on top.

Combine all sauce ingredients in saucepan, bring to boil, and lower heat. Simmer, stirring frequently, for 25 minutes. Pour sauce over chicken mixture and bake in 350° F. oven for 1 hour.

Serves 2.

MANICOTTI WITH CHICKEN AND SPINACH

(3 fat units per serving)

    1 large chicken breast, skinned
    ¼ cup chopped onions
    2 or 3 cloves garlic, minced
    ¾ cup cooked chopped and drained spinach
    ¼ cup low fat cottage cheese
    1 teaspoon nutmeg
    4 ounces manicotti

CREAM SAUCE:

    2 cups skim milk
    1 tablespoon arrowroot
    2 tablespoons chicken stock (see page 118)
    Pepper and salt to taste

Poach chicken in water for about 20 minutes. Cool. Strip meat and cut into small slivers. Sauté onion and garlic in a nonstick frying pan. Stir until soft. Add spinach, cottage cheese, chicken and nutmeg. Set aside.

Parboil manicotti according to package directions. Do not overcook, or manicotti will split. Drain. Fill each with chicken mixture and place in a shallow 2-quart pyrex dish.

(Continued)

To make sauce, combine milk, arrowroot, chicken stock, and pepper and salt in saucepan. Stir over low heat with wire whisk until sauce thickens, about 15 minutes. Pour sauce over manicotti, sprinkle with additional nutmeg, and bake in a 350° F. oven for 25 minutes.

Serves 2.

ORIENTAL SHRIMP AND NOODLES

(½ fat unit per serving)

¼ cup chopped onions
1 large green pepper, cut into strips
⅓ cup undiluted frozen unsweetened orange-juice concentrate
¼ cup water
3 tablespoons vinegar
1 teaspoon curry powder
1 tablespoon soy sauce
¾ cup chopped green onion tops
6 ounces shrimp, cleaned
2 cups cooked green noodles

Cook onion and green pepper in a nonstick skillet, over low heat, until vegetables are soft, about 10 minutes. Combine orange juice, water, vinegar, curry powder and soy sauce; add to skillet. Add shrimp and green onion tops; cook until shrimp turns pink, about 5 minutes. Serve over cooked green noodles.

Serves 2.

VEGETABLE DISHES

STUFFED GREEN PEPPERS

(1 fat unit per serving)

2 medium green peppers
⅔ cup chicken stock (see page 118)
⅓ cup bulgur wheat

3 tablespoons minced mushroom
¼ cup minced onion
¼ cup minced celery
½ teaspoon caraway seeds
1 tablespoon undiluted frozen unsweetened orange-juice
    concentrate
Black pepper and salt to taste

Cut a slice, including stem, from the top of each green pepper. Remove stems; mince the slices and set aside. Clean out seeds from peppers and rinse. Drop peppers into a saucepan of boiling water; parboil for 5 minutes. Remove and let drain upside down.

Bring chicken stock to a boil; stir in bulgur wheat. Lower heat and simmer until liquid has been absorbed. Remove from heat.

In a nonstick skillet, combine reserved minced green pepper, mushrooms, onion and celery; sauté, stirring constantly, for 5 minutes. Remove from heat, add caraway seeds and orange-juice concentrate; stir into bulgur wheat mixture and add salt and pepper. Stuff peppers with mixture. Place in a small pan with 1 inch of water. Bake in a preheated 350° F. oven for 40 minutes.

Serves 2.

POTATO SOUFFLÉ

(1 fat unit per serving)

2½ cups grated potatoes (about 2 baking potatoes)
1 egg yolk
1 teaspoon dry hot mustard
2 tablespoons flour
Black pepper and salt to taste
3 egg whites
1 teaspoon paprika

Combine potatoes, egg yolk, mustard, flour, and pepper and salt. Beat egg whites until stiff peaks form; fold into potato mixture. Pour into a small casserole. Sprinkle with paprika. Bake in a 375° F. oven 40–45 minutes. Serve at once.

Serves 2.

RATATOUILLE

(1 fat unit per serving)

1 cup peeled and diced eggplant
2 cloves garlic, minced
1¼ cups chicken stock (see page 118)
Salt and pepper to taste
Juice of 1 lemon
½ cup green pepper strips
½ cup sliced mushrooms
½ cup sliced onion
½ cup diced yellow squash
¼ teaspoon mace
¾ cup canned tomatoes, drained
1 teaspoon basil

Place eggplant, half the minced garlic, and ¼ cup of the chicken stock in a heavy pot. Add salt and pepper. Bring to a boil; lower heat and simmer 10–15 minutes, or until eggplant has absorbed stock and is tender. Place eggplant in the bottom of a small baking dish, sprinkle with some lemon juice, and set aside.

Cook the green pepper strips, the rest of the garlic, and ¼ cup of the chicken stock, until all liquid has been absorbed, about 10 minutes; layer over the eggplant and sprinkle with lemon juice.

Cook the mushrooms and onions with ¼ cup of chicken stock until all liquid has been absorbed, about 8 minutes; spoon over eggplant and peppers, and sprinkle with lemon juice.

Place squash in a saucepan with ¼ cup chicken stock; cook for 10 minutes with mace, salt and pepper. Add squash to casserole and sprinkle with lemon juice. Add the tomatoes, basil and remaining ¼ cup of chicken stock. Sprinkle with lemon juice, salt and pepper. Bake in a 350° F. oven for 15 minutes, or until hot. Serve at once or chill and serve cold.

Serves 2 as a vegetable, or 4 as an appetizer.

REFRIED BEANS

(½ fat unit per serving)

2 cups cooked kidney beans
¾ cup finely chopped onions
¼ cup chicken stock (see page 118)

¼ cup canned tomatoes, with juice
2 cloves garlic, minced
½ teaspoon ground celery seed
1 tablespoon lemon juice
5 drops Tabasco
Black pepper and salt to taste

Combine all ingredients in a nonstick skillet. Simmer, covered, over low heat about 50–60 minutes, until beans are dry and all liquid has been absorbed. Serve hot.

Serves 2.

STEAMED SPINACH WITH NUTMEG

(0 fat units per recipe)

1 pound fresh spinach leaves
½ teaspoon ground nutmeg
Salt and pepper to taste

Wash and trim spinach leaves. Place into a steamer over boiling water. Sprinkle with nutmeg, salt and pepper. Cover tightly and steam for 10 minutes, or until spinach is just wilted.

Serves 4.

NO-FAT FRENCH FRIES

(0 fat units per serving)

2 medium-size baking potatoes
Salt
Pepper

Peel potatoes. Cut into strips the length of the potato and about ⅛- to ¼-inch thick. Spread the potatoes in a single layer on a cookie sheet or shallow baking pan. Salt the potatoes and bake in a hot 400° F. oven about 1 hour. Sprinkle with black pepper and serve.

Serves 2.

SCALLOPED POTATOES PARMESAN

(1½ fat units per recipe)

2 medium baking potatoes
1 cup skim milk
Salt and pepper to taste
1 tablespoon grated Parmesan cheese

Wash and peel the potatoes; cut into thin slices. Place a layer of potato slices in a nonstick pie pan, pour in just enough milk to cover. Add a sprinkling of salt and pepper and 1 teaspoon grated Parmesan cheese. Add a second and a third layer of potatoes, milk, salt, pepper and grated Parmesan cheese. Cover with foil and bake in a 375° F. oven for 30 minutes. Remove the foil and continue to bake until the potatoes are tender when pierced with a fork and the top layer is lightly browned.

Serves 2.

TOPPINGS FOR BAKED POTATOES

(½ fat unit per each recipe)

CHEESE TOPPING:
⅓ cup low fat cottage cheese
2 tablespoons minced green pepper
1 tablespoon minced onion
¼ teaspoon curry powder
Black pepper and salt to taste

Combine all ingredients; stir well. Refrigerate until ready to use.

YOGURT ONION TOPPING:
⅓ cup low fat plain yogurt
3 tablespoons minced green onion
¼ teaspoon dry horseradish
Black pepper and salt to taste

Combine all ingredients; stir well. Refrigerate until ready to use.

CUCUMBER DILL TOPPING:
⅓ cup low fat plain yogurt
¼ cup minced cucumber

1 teaspoon lemon juice
¼ teaspoon dill weed
Black pepper and salt to taste

Combine all ingredients; stir well. Refrigerate until ready to use.

MUSHROOM YOGURT TOPPING:
    ¼ cup mushrooms
    3 tablespoons minced onion
    ½ teaspoon tarragon
    ⅓ cup low fat plain yogurt

Sauté mushrooms and onions in a small nonstick skillet, until mushrooms are soft and dark, about 5 minutes. Add tarragon and stir in yogurt. Refrigerate until ready to use.

VEGETABLE PATÉ

(½ fat unit per recipe)

1 cup broccoli, cut in flowerets
2 cups spinach, tightly packed
1 cup mushrooms
⅓ cup minced onion
3 cloves garlic, minced
1 teaspoon nutmeg
Juice of ½ lemon
½ cup low fat cottage cheese
2 egg whites
2 teaspoons curry powder
Salt and pepper to taste
Paprika

Simmer broccoli in a little water or steam until cooked tender. Drain and set aside. Simmer spinach in a little water until soft, about 2 minutes; drain and set aside. Sauté mushrooms, onion and garlic in a nonstick skillet, until soft. Place a layer of spinach in a nonstick pan; sprinkle with nutmeg and squeeze lemon juice over it.

Beat egg whites until stiff.

In an electric blender, mix cottage cheese, egg whites, curry powder, salt and pepper; pour ⅓ of this mixture over the spinach. Top with the mushroom mixture; then another ⅓ of the cheese

(Continued)

mixture; then with the cooked broccoli, and finally with the remaining cheese mixture. Sprinkle with salt, pepper and paprika. Set the pan into a larger pan that contains about 1 inch of water. Bake in a 375° F. oven for 1 hour. Serve at room temperature.

Serves 2.

SALADS

POTATO SALAD

(½ fat unit per serving)

3 medium-size potatoes
⅓ cup chicken stock (see page 118)
¼ cup low fat plain yogurt
3 tablespoons minced green pepper
1 hard-boiled egg white, diced
⅓ cup minced onion
¼ teaspoon celery seed
¼ teaspoon dill weed
Black pepper and salt to taste
1 tablespoon minced parsley

Boil potatoes until tender. Peel while hot, slice, and immediately combine with all other ingredients. Chill. Before serving, sprinkle with minced parsley.

Serves 2.

KIDNEY BEAN SALAD

(½ fat unit per serving)

2 cups cooked kidney beans
1 cup cooked green beans, cut into small pieces
½ cup minced green onions, including tops
¼ cup minced green pepper
3 tablespoons minced celery
2 cloves garlic, minced
2 teaspoons capers
½ teaspoon cilantro (coriander leaves)

Black pepper and salt to taste
6 tablespoons Tomato Salad Dressing (see page 119)
1 tablespoon chopped parsley

Combine all ingredients except parsley. Refrigerate for at least 3 hours. Sprinkle with parsley before serving.

Serves 4.

RICE SALAD

(½ fat unit per serving)

1½ cups cooked white long-grained rice
½ cup cooked green peas
½ cup cooked cut green beans
¼ cup finely chopped cucumber
1 hard-boiled egg white, chopped
½ cup minced green onion, including tops
2 tablespoons minced green pepper
2 tablespoons minced celery
1 tablespoon tarragon
Black pepper and salt to taste
6 tablespoons Tomato Salad Dressing (see page 119)

Combine all ingredients and chill for at least 3 hours.

Serves 4.

LENTIL SALAD

(0 fat units per serving)

2 cups lentils, cooked but firm
2 cups sliced carrots, cooked but firm
½ cup chopped celery
½ cup minced green onion, including tops
½ cup minced onion
1 cup finely chopped raw cabbage
1 clove garlic, minced
1 teaspoon ground celery seed
1 tablespoon Hungarian sweet paprika
Black pepper and salt to taste
1 cup Tomato Salad Dressing (see page 119)

Combine all ingredients. Chill.

Serves 6.

TURNIP SLAW

(0 fat units per serving)

2 cups peeled and grated raw white turnip
¼ cup grated onion
1 chopped apple, with peel, preferably tart
1 tablespoon undiluted frozen unsweetened orange-juice
    concentrate
1 tablespoon lemon juice
½ teaspoon whole celery seed
½ teaspoon caraway seed
Black pepper and salt to taste
½ cup Tart Banana Dressing (see page 120)

Combine all ingredients. Refrigerate for at least 3 hours, or preferably overnight.

Serves 2.

COLE SLAW

(½ fat unit per recipe)

4 cups shredded cabbage
½ cup grated carrot
½ cup finely minced green pepper
¼ cup thinly sliced onion
1 cup low fat plain yogurt
2 tablespoons undiluted frozen unsweetened apple-juice
    concentrate
1 tablespoon tarragon vinegar
1 teaspoon celery seed

Combine cabbage, carrot, green pepper and onion in a large bowl. Stir together the yogurt, apple-juice concentrate, tarragon vinegar and celery seed; pour over the cabbage mixture and toss lightly to coat well. Refrigerate for several hours to allow flavors to blend.

Serves 6.

BEET SALAD

(0 fat units per serving)

1 bunch watercress, washed, stems removed
3 large cooked beets, sliced
1 small orange, thinly sliced
1 small onion, thinly sliced
¼ cup Tomato Salad Dressing (see page 119)

Cover two salad plates with the watercress. Arrange slices of beet, orange and onion. (You may wish to soak the onion in cold water for about 45 minutes before adding to salad, to lessen the strong flavor.) Spoon Tomato Salad Dressing over just before serving.

Serves 4.

CHESTNUT WALDORF SALAD

(0 fat units per serving)

1 cup diced unpeeled apple
Juice of ½ lemon
½ cup sliced water chestnuts
½ cup sliced bananas, dipped in lemon juice
½ cup diced celery
½ cup Tart Banana Dressing (see page 120)
2 tablespoons minced parsley

Combine apple, lemon juice, water chestnuts, banana and celery. Stir in ⅓ cup dressing and 1 tablespoon of parsley; refrigerate. Before serving, add rest of dressing and sprinkle remaining parsley on top.

Serves 2.

DESSERTS

APPLE CRUNCH

(1 fat unit per serving)

1 large tart apple
Juice of 1 lemon
½ teaspoon cinnamon
1 pear
½ teaspoon ground allspice
1 cup French bread cubes
½ teaspoon ground coriander
2 tablespoons Grape Nuts cereal
½ cup low fat plain yogurt
3 tablespoons undiluted frozen unsweetened orange-juice
    concentrate
1 teaspoon vanilla

Peel and dice apple; place slices in a small casserole and squeeze juice of ½ lemon over it. Sprinkle with cinnamon. Peel and cut up pear. Place slices over apple and squeeze remaining ½ lemon over it. Sprinkle with allspice, top with bread cubes, and sprinkle with coriander.

Bake in a 375° F. oven for about 20 minutes. Remove from oven and sprinkle with Grape Nuts. Serve with sauce made by combining yogurt, orange-juice concentrate and vanilla; stir until smooth.

Serves 2.

BANANA WHIP

(0 fat units per serving)

2 egg whites
2 small ripe bananas
3 tablespoons undiluted frozen unsweetened orange-juice
    concentrate
1 teaspoon almond extract
1 teaspoon nutmeg
½ teaspoon grated lemon rind

Beat egg whites until stiff but not dry. Set aside. Mash bananas. Add other ingredients and beat with an electric mixer until mixture is thick and smooth. Fold in egg whites. Spoon into two tall parfait glasses. Chill for several hours. About 45 minutes before serving, put parfaits in the freezer.

Serves 2.

BAKED FRUIT

(½ fat unit per serving)

2 cups of any of the following fruits, alone or in combination:
rhubarb, chopped
apples, peeled and chopped
pears, peeled and chopped
peaches, peeled and sliced
blueberries, cleaned, stems removed
1 tablespoon honey
1 tablespoon lemon juice
½ teaspoon cinnamon
½ teaspoon cardamom

Place fruit in a small casserole. Add honey and mix through. Sprinkle with lemon juice, sprinkle with spices. Bake about 20 minutes in a 350° F. oven. Serve warm or cold.

Serves 2.

CHEESE DESSERT

(3 fat units per serving)

1 cup low fat cottage cheese
1 large egg
6 tablespoons orange juice
¼ cup low fat plain yogurt
2 tablespoons honey
1 tablespoon bread crumbs
1 teaspoon nutmeg

Blend cheese, egg, juice, yogurt and honey in an electric blender until mixture is thick and smooth. Pour into a small casserole or two individual ramekins. Mix bread crumbs and nutmeg and sprinkle on top. Bake in a 350° F. oven 35–40 minutes. Chill.

Serves 2.

PUMPKIN PUDDING

(2½ fat units per serving)

3 egg whites
1¼ cups plain pumpkin, fresh or canned
½ cup low fat plain yogurt
6 tablespoons undiluted frozen unsweetened orange-juice concentrate
2 tablespoons honey
1½ teaspoons cinnamon
1 teaspoon ground allspice

Beat egg whites until stiff but not dry. Combine all other ingredients; fold egg whites into mixture. Pour into a casserole. Bake in a 350° F. oven 45–50 minutes. Chill before serving.

Serves 2.

PLUM PUDDING

(½ fat unit per serving)

2 cups unpeeled plums, cut up
Juice of ½ lemon
3 tablespoons bread crumbs
1 teaspoon anise seed

SAUCE:

½ cup low fat plain yogurt
6 tablespoons undiluted frozen unsweetened apple-juice concentrate
1 tablespoon flour
2 teaspoons ground coriander

Place cut plums in a casserole dish or in individual ramekins. Squeeze lemon juice over plums. To make sauce, combine all ingredients in a mixing bowl and beat well with a wire whisk until thoroughly blended. Pour sauce over fruit. Mix bread crumbs and anise seed; sprinkle mixture over fruit. Bake, uncovered, in a 350° F. oven for 30 minutes. Serve warm or chilled.

Serves 2.

FRUIT CUP

(0 fat units per serving)

Combine two or more of the following fruits to equal 2½ cups:
grapes, seedless
orange or tangerine segments
cantaloupe balls
pears, peeled and sliced and dipped in lemon juice
bananas, sliced and dipped in lemon juice

SAUCE:
1 cup cut-up cantaloupe or bananas
1 teaspoon vanilla

Spoon fruit into two parfait glasses. Purée cantaloupe or bananas and vanilla in an electric blender to make sauce. Pour over fruit; refrigerate. About 45 minutes before serving, place parfaits in freezer.

Serves 2.

FRUIT SHERBET

(0 fat units per serving)

1 large banana
1 large navel orange
1 teaspoon vanilla
½ cup water
2 egg whites

Blend fruit, vanilla and water in an electric blender. Beat egg whites until stiff but not dry; fold into fruit mixture. Pour into a shallow pan or bowl; place in freezer until mixture is solid around the edges but still soft in the middle. Remove from freezer and beat until smooth. Return to freezer. When partially frozen, remove and beat again until smooth. Pour into two parfait glasses. Freeze until firm.

Before serving, garnish with a few purple grapes or wedges of tangerine. If desired, about 10 minutes before serving, place glasses in refrigerator to soften sherbet a bit.

Serves 2.

BAKED APPLES

(0 fat units per serving)

2 large tart baking apples, unpeeled
1 tablespoon lemon juice
Nutmeg

SAUCE:

½ cup undiluted frozen unsweetened apple-juice concentrate
3 tablespoons lemon juice or orange juice
3 tablespoons water
1 teaspoon arrowroot

Wash and core apples. Sprinkle lemon juice into cavities and sprinkle with nutmeg. Set apples in a small baking pan with 1 inch of water. Bake in a 325° F. oven for 45 minutes, or longer if you prefer softer apples.

Combine sauce ingredients in a saucepan; simmer, stirring constantly, until slightly thickened. Remove from heat, pour over apples, and serve warm.

Serves 2.

BAKED BANANAS

(0 fat units per serving)

2 peeled and cored tart apples, cut in half
2 teaspoons cinnamon
2 bananas
2 tablespoons Grape Nuts
2 teaspoons lemon juice

Place apples in a saucepan, cover with water and add 1 teaspoon cinnamon; cook until soft. Slice bananas in half lengthwise. Place in a shallow casserole and sprinkle with remaining cinnamon. Top bananas with cooked apple; sprinkle with Grape Nuts and lemon juice. Bake in a 375° F. oven for 10 minutes. Then put under the broiler for 5 minutes more.

Serves 2.

FRUIT AND RICE MERINGUE

(0 fat units per serving)

1 cup cooked brown rice
½ cup unsweetened pineapple chunks
1 pear, peeled and sliced
Juice of ½ lemon
¼ cup undiluted unsweetened frozen apple-juice concentrate
¼ cup water
3 egg whites

Place rice in a small casserole; top with pineapple and pear. Squeeze lemon juice over fruit. Add apple-juice concentrate mixed with water. Bake in a 350° F. oven for 20 minutes.

Meanwhile, beat egg whites until stiff peaks form. Drop spoonfuls over top of dessert, covering the fruit. Bake for an additional 10 to 15 minutes in a 350° F. oven, until meringue has browned.

Serves 2.

BREADS

GINGER MUFFINS

(2 fat units per recipe)

2 or 3 ripe bananas (1 cup mashed)
3 egg whites
1 cup whole wheat flour
1½ teaspoons baking powder
1 teaspoon baking soda
2 tablespoons undiluted frozen unsweetened orange-juice
    concentrate
½ cup low fat plain yogurt
1 teaspoon ginger
1 teaspoon nutmeg
1 tablespoon honey

(Continued)

Mash or purée the bananas. Beat egg whites until foamy and thick. Sift flour, baking powder and baking soda into a large bowl. Add bananas, orange juice, yogurt, ginger, nutmeg and honey. Mix well. Stir beaten egg whites into batter; pour mixture into nonstick muffin pans. Bake about 30 minutes in a 350° F. oven.

Makes 12 muffins, 2½ inches in diameter.

SQUASH BREAD

(2 fat units per recipe)

    1 cup whole wheat flour
    1½ teaspoons baking powder
    1 teaspon baking soda
    1 cup grated raw yellow squash
    ½ cup low fat plain yogurt
    2 teaspoons lemon juice
    1 teaspoon cinnamon
    1 teaspoon mace
    2 tablespoons honey
    3 egg whites

Sift flour, baking powder and baking soda into a large bowl. Add squash, then all other ingredients except egg whites. Beat egg whites until foamy. Stir into batter. Pour batter into a pan, 8x8x2-inch. Bake in a 350° F. oven for 30 minutes.

Makes 1 loaf of bread.

APPLE OATMEAL LOAF

(2 fat units per recipe)

    3 cups peeled tart apples
    ¾ cup unsifted whole wheat flour
    ½ cup oatmeal, uncooked
    3 tablespoons ground cinnamon
    ¼ cup undiluted frozen unsweetened orange-juice concentrate
    ½ cup buttermilk
    ¼ cup low fat plain yogurt
    1 teaspoon vanilla
    3 egg whites

Slice apples to fill ¾ of a cup, then chop the remaining 2¾ cups. Combine chopped apples with remaining ingredients except for egg whites. Beat egg whites until stiff peaks form; fold into batter. Pour batter into a 9-inch round nonstick cake pan. Arrange reserved apple slices over the top. Sprinkle with additional cinnamon. Bake in a 350° F. oven for about 1 hour. Serve warm.

Serves 8.

CORN BREAD

(2 fat units per recipe)

1 cup whole wheat flour
1 cup cornmeal, white or yellow
1 tablespoon double-acting baking powder
1 cup low fat plain yogurt
½ cup tomato juice
¼ cup undiluted frozen unsweetened orange-juice concentrate
2 egg whites

Sift together whole wheat flour, cornmeal and baking powder. Add yogurt, tomato juice and orange-juice concentrate. Beat egg whites until foamy; add to batter. Pour into a nonstick 8x8x2-inch pan. Bake in a 350° F. oven for 40 minutes, or until toothpick inserted into middle comes out clean. Serve warm.

Serves 8.

SAUCES, STOCKS and DRESSINGS

FISH SAUCE

(½ fat unit per recipe)

½ cup low fat plain yogurt
1 tablespoon minced green pepper
1 tablespoon minced onion
2 tablespoons minced cucumber
1 teaspoon capers
2 teaspoons lemon juice
¼ teaspoon paprika
Black pepper and salt to taste

Combine all ingredients. Chill for at least 1 hour.

Makes about ¾ cup.

CHICKEN OR TURKEY STOCK

(1 fat unit per cup)

3 pounds chicken necks and backs, or turkey wings
3 quarts water
1 whole onion
3 stalks celery
2 carrots, scraped and halved
2 bay leaves
1 tablespoon whole black peppercorns
1 tablespoon thyme
2 cloves garlic, optional
Few sprigs parsley

Bring all ingredients to a boil in a large saucepan. Simmer over very low heat for about 3½ hours. Skim surface from time to time, to remove fat. When done, strain stock and put into a bowl. Refrigerate overnight. Before using or freezing, skim off all fat which will have risen to the surface. Keep refrigerated.

Makes about 2 quarts.

VEGETABLE STOCK

(0 fat units per recipe)

2 quarts water
½ medium onion
2 carrots
2 stalks celery
2 parsnips
1 small turnip
Black pepper to taste

Combine all ingredients in a large saucepan. Bring to a boil, lower heat and simmer for 1 hour. Skim occasionally. Strain, mashing vegetables to extract all liquid. Discard vegetables and use stock as needed. Keep refrigerated.

Makes about 1½ quarts.

TOMATO SALAD DRESSING

(0 fat units per tablespoon)

1 17-ounce can tomatoes, with juice
¾ cup chopped onion
2 tablespoons chopped celery
2 cloves garlic, minced
1 teaspoon basil
1 teaspoon dry hot mustard
1 teaspoon lemon juice
Black pepper to taste
⅓ cup water

Combine all ingredients; bring to a boil, then lower heat and simmer for 30 minutes. Purée in an electric blender. Chill.

Makes about 2⅓ cups.

NOTE: This recipe can be used in a variety of ways. If vinegar is added to it, the dressing will be nippier. Use it as a sauce for baked chicken or fish. Add spice, Tabasco sauce, a few drops of Worcestershire sauce and some celery seed; chill and serve as a cocktail.

TART BANANA DRESSING

(0 fat units per recipe)

1 medium banana
1 small onion, chopped
2 tablespoons undiluted frozen unsweetened apple-juice
      concentrate
6 drops Tabasco
Black pepper to taste

Purée ingredients in an electric blender. Refrigerate.

Makes about 1¼ cups dressing.

TANGY BOILED DRESSING

(3 fat units per recipe)

1 egg plus 1 egg white
1 teaspoon hot dry mustard
1 tablespoon vinegar
Salt and pepper to taste
½ cup low fat plain yogurt
½ cup skim milk
2½ teaspoons arrowroot

Combine egg and egg white, mustard, vinegar, salt and pepper in an electric blender. Blend for a few seconds at high speed, then lower speed and slowly add the yogurt, milk and arrowroot. Pour mixture into a saucepan. Simmer over low heat, stirring constantly, until thickened. Chill. Whip just before serving.

Makes about 1¼ cups.

MOCK SOUR CREAM

(1½ fat units per recipe)

1 cup low fat cottage cheese
1 cup low fat plain yogurt
2 teaspoons cider vinegar

Place all ingredients into an electric blender; process on high until mixture is smooth and thick. Refrigerate.

Makes 2 cups.

CRANBERRY RELISH

(0 fat units per recipe)

1 cup cranberries, rinsed, drained, stems removed
5 tablespoons undiluted frozen unsweetened orange-juice
    concentrate
1 tablespoon lemon juice
½ cup peeled and chopped pear
1 tablespoon water
¼ teaspoon ground cloves
¼ teaspoon ground cinnamon
¼ teaspoon ground coriander

Combine all ingredients in a saucepan. Bring to a boil over high heat, then lower heat and simmer for 15 minutes. Chill before serving.

Makes 1 cup.

PICKLED FRUIT RELISH*

(0 fat units per recipe)

½ cup vinegar
6 tablespoons undiluted frozen unsweetened orange-juice
    concentrate
¼ cup water
1 2-inch stick cinnamon
8 whole cloves
½ teaspoon allspice
1 peach, peeled, quartered, and pitted
1 pear, peeled, core removed, and quartered
2 plums, peeled, cut in half, pitted

Combine vinegar, orange juice and water in a heavy saucepan. Stir with a wire whisk until thoroughly blended. Add cinnamon, cloves and allspice; simmer for 15 minutes. Add fruit; bring mixture to a boil, lower heat and simmer for an additional 15 minutes. Refrigerate fruits in liquid; drain fruits before serving.

Makes about 1 cup.

* Pickled fruit relish is excellent when served with meat or poultry. Juice remaining after the fruit is removed can be used again.

CREAM SAUCE

(2 fat units per recipe)

2 cups skim milk
1 tablespoon arrowroot
2 tablespoons chicken stock (see page 118)
Salt and pepper to taste

Stir all ingredients over low heat, with a wire whisk, until sauce thickens, about 15 minutes. This flavorful sauce, so simple to make, can be used to cream chicken or turkey, or used as a sauce for vegetables or noodles.

Makes 2 cups.

ORANGE DRESSING*

(1 fat unit per recipe)

1 cup chicken stock (see page 000)
⅓ cup undiluted frozen unsweetened orange-juice concentrate
1 teaspoon rosemary
2 teaspoons arrowroot
Pepper to taste

Combine chicken stock, orange-juice concentrate, rosemary, arrowroot and pepper. Beat with a wire whisk. Bring to a boil, then immediately lower heat and simmer, stirring constantly, until sauce has thickened. Chill.

Makes about 1 cup.

MUSTARD SAUCE

(½ fat unit per recipe)

½ cup low fat plain yogurt
1 teaspoon Dijon mustard
Salt and pepper to taste

Combine all ingredients. Chill until ready to use.

Makes ½ cup.

---

* Sauce may be used over cold chicken, turkey or fruit.

HORSERADISH SAUCE

(0 fat units per recipe)

½ cup undiluted frozen unsweetened apple-juice concentrate
2 tablespoons vinegar
1 teaspoon dry horseradish
A few shakes of cayenne pepper

Combine all ingredients and stir to mix thoroughly.

Makes ½ cup.

TARRAGON SAUCE

(½ fat unit per recipe)

½ cup tarragon vinegar
1½ cups canned tomatoes, with juice
¼ cup chopped onions
½ cup low fat plain yogurt
¼ cup sliced mushrooms
1 teaspoon chili powder
Black pepper and salt to taste

Combine all ingredients in a saucepan; bring to a boil, then lower heat and simmer, stirring frequently, for 25 minutes.

Makes about 3 cups.

SAUCE FOR SPAGHETTI

(4½ fat units per recipe with beef)
(¼ fat unit per recipe without beef)

4 ounces ground lean beef
1 17-ounce can tomatoes, with juice
⅔ cup chopped onions
½ cup sliced mushrooms
⅓ cup chopped green pepper
2 cloves garlic, minced
¼ cup chicken stock (see page 118)
2 tablespoons minced parsley
1½ teaspoons oregano
¼ teaspoon ground cloves
1 teaspoon basil
2 teaspoons lemon juice
Black pepper and salt to taste

(Continued)

Brown meat in a nonstick skillet; drain off any fat that accumulates. Add all vegetables and seasonings and chicken stock; bring to a boil. Lower heat and simmer for 25 minutes.

Makes about 3 cups.

TUNA SAUCE

(2 fat units per recipe)

2 cups canned tomatoes, drained
1 cup chopped onions
½ cup diced green pepper
½ cup minced celery
3 cloves garlic, minced
1½ teaspoons basil
1 7-ounce can solid pack tuna, waterpacked
½ cup tomato juice (use juice from tomatoes)

Place tomatoes in a heavy skillet or Dutch oven. Add onions, pepper, celery, garlic and basil. Simmer 20–25 minutes. Add tuna, drained and broken up. Add tomato juice. Simmer only until mixture is heated through. Serve over spaghetti or other pasta, cooked al dente.

Makes about 4 cups.

PART III

THE FAT UNITS COUNTER

How to Count Fat Units
to Shed Pounds

This counter—the only one of its kind—shows how easily you can keep to 7 fat units a day and watch that weight disappear.

The Following Charts Are Indispensable:

Listed in this section are more than 2,500 food items and drinks listed with their appropriate fat units. To lose excess weight, eat as much as you like of the foods which are given a 0 rating on the chart. Restrict all foods which are given a fat unit count so that you do not consume more than 7 units of fat in total in any one day.

The 7-Unit Fat Counter is the essential tool in your plan to lose weight and lose it permanently. Generic foods (meats, vegetables, fruits, etc.) are unit counted, as well as the most popular brand name convenience foods. You'll find among these convenience foods many choices for well-balanced one-dish meals, breads and cake mixes, soups, low-cal salad dressings, and so on, within this guide. We've even unit counted foods served in the best-known fast food chains. Thus, in addition to the 111 recipes provided in the recipe section, you are provided with hundreds of ways to prepare delicious, nutritious low fat meals.

In case you don't find the fat units for a certain food in the list that follows—and you know the number of fat grams in the food (which sometimes appears on food labels)—you can convert them to fat units. Here's how:

> 1 fat unit equals 2.835 fat grams.
> So, if an ounce of food has 2 grams of fat, you divide 2 by 2.8. The answer is .75, which you can round off to 1 fat unit.

> Another example:
> If 3 ounces of a food have 10 grams of fat you divide by 2.8 and get 3½ fat units.

The fat units, in almost all cases, reflect the absolute fat content of foods. But in some cases, they have been adjusted slightly up or down at the authors' discretion to account for higher sugar or caloric content or higher bulk of certain foods, in keeping with the theory of this diet.

Free foods: Among the foods given 0 fat unit ratings are fresh fruit, vegetables, pasta and rice. You can consume these foods freely. *You need restrict them only if they are cooked or served with fat, in which case you should count the appropriate fat units for the amount of fat or oil used.*

Sweet foods and drinks: Some sweet foods, such as jellies and soft drinks, do not have fat but do add up to large numbers of calories that could ruin your diet. Thus, we have given them equivalent fat-unit ratings.

Alcohol: If you want to drink a moderate amount of alcohol (one drink a day) while dieting, you can. But, of course, as mentioned earlier, excessive consumption would retard weight loss. (See page 10)

Fat-Free but High-Calorie Sweet Foods and Soft Drinks

Naturally sweet foods like fresh fruit are allowed in unlimited quantities on this diet. Many other sweet foods have a fat content and you will find them in the main lists. The following very sweet foods are fat-free, but high calorie. To ensure that, if you eat them, you do not exceed your correct dieting intake, we suggest that you subtract the following equivalent units from your daily allowance of 7:

	Equivalent Fat Units
Candy, hard and mint: 1 oz.	4
Cranberry sauce: ½ cup	8
Dried fruits, all types: 1 oz.	2
Fruit, canned in heavy syrup: ½ cup	3
Gelatin, sweetened: ½ cup	3
Jams, jellies, preserves, marmalade	
regular: 1 tbsp	1½
low calorie: 1 tbsp	1
Juices, fruit, sweetened or fruit drinks: 4 oz.	2½
Marshmallows, regular size: 1	1
Soft drinks: 8 fl. oz.	
Colas	4
Diet colas	0
Club soda	0

	Equivalent Fat Units
Fruit flavored	4½
Collins mixer	3½
Bitter lemon	4
Ginger ale	3½
Iced tea, sweetened	5
Root beer	4½
Tonic water	3½
Sugar or honey: 1 tbsp	2
Toppings and syrups: 1 tbsp	2½
Toppings, no calorie	0

Alcoholic Drinks

Distilled liquor: 1½ fl. oz. (1 jigger)
Whiskey, gin, rum, vodka, tequila, unflavored brandy:

	Equivalent Fat Units
70 proof	3
80 proof	3½
86 proof	4
90 proof	4½
94 proof	4½
100 proof	5

Wines and apéritifs: 1 fl. oz.:

Campari	2½
Cinzano	2
Dubonnet, dry	1½
Dubonnet, red	2
Sherry, dry	1
Sherry, medium	1½
Sherry, cream	1½
Port, all types	1½
Vermouth, dry	1½
White, dry	1

	Equivalent Fat Units
White, sparkling	1
White, sweet	1½
Rosé	1
Wine, red, dry	1
Wine, red, sweet	1½
Wine, rosé	1

Beer: 12 fl. oz.:

Regular	6
Light	4

GENERIC FOODS

			Fat Units

BREAD
All kinds: white, wheat, rye, pumpernickel, pita, 1 oz. or 1 regular size slice ½

BUTTER

Regular: ½ cup	33	Whipped: ½ cup	21½
Regular: 1 tbsp	4	Whipped: 1 tbsp	3

CHEESES   1 oz. unless noted

American, processed	3	Muenster	3
Blue	3	Neufchatel	2½
Brick	3	Parmesan	3
Brie	3	Port du Salut	3
Camembert	2½	Provolone	2½
Caraway	3	Ricotta, whole milk: 1 cup	11½
Cheddar	3½	Ricotta, partially skim milk:	
Cheshire	3	1 cup	7
Colby	3	Romano	2½
Edam	3	Roquefort	3
Farmer	1	Swiss, natural	3
Feta	2	Swiss, processed	2½
Fontina	3	Tilsit	2½
Gjetost	3	Cottage cheese	
Gouda	3	Regular: ½ cup	2
Gruyère	3½	Dry, pot style: ½ cup	½
Limburger	2½	Low fat: ½ cup	½
Monterey	3	Cream cheese: 1 oz.	3½
Mozzarella	2	Cream cheese, imitation: 1 oz.	1½
Mozzarella, low moisture	2½	Cheese food: 1 oz.	2½
Mozzarella, part skim	1½	Cheese spread: 1 oz.	2
Mozzarella, low moisture, part skim	1½		

COCONUT

Meat: 1 piece, 2x2x½″	5½	Meat, shredded or grated: ¼ cup	2½

COFFEE   0

CORNSTARCH   0

CREAM   1 tbsp

Medium cream (25% fat)	1½	Heavy whipping cream	
Light cream	1	(unwhipped)	2
Half-and-half	½	Light whipping cream	
Sour cream	1	(unwhipped)	1½
Whipped cream topping	½		

Fat Units

EGGS 1

Extra large	2½	Yolk only, large, extra large	2
Large, medium	2	White only	0

FISH, Fresh, Raw   3 oz. unless noted

Anchovy	½	Rabbitfish, fillet	½
Bass, striped, fillet	½	Rockfish, fillet	½
Carp, fillet	1½	Sablefish, fillet	4
Catfish, channel, fillet	1	Salmon, fillet or steak	2
Caviar: 1 oz.	1½	Sea bass	1
1 tbsp	1	Shad, fillet	½
Cod, fillet	½	Smelt, rainbow	½
Eel	5½	Snapper, red, fillet	½
Flounder fillet	½	Sole, fillet	½
Haddock, fillet	½	Sprat, fillet	1
Hake, fillet	½	Sturgeon, fillet	1
Halibut	½	Trout, rainbow, fillet	1½
Herring, fillet	2	Trout, brook, whole eviscerated	2½
Mackerel, Atlantic, fillet	3	Tuna, albacore, white meat	2½
Mullet, striped	2	Turbot	2½
Ocean perch, fillet	½	Whitefish, lake, fillet	1½
Pike, northern, fillet	½	Yellowtail, fillet	1½

FLOUR

Buckwheat: 1 cup	½	Low fat: 1 cup	2
Carob: 1 cup	½	Defatted: 1 cup	½
Corn: 1 cup	1	Wheat:	
Peanut flour, defatted: 1 cup	2	All purpose: 1 cup	½
Rye: 1 cup	½	Whole wheat and gluten:	
Soybean:		1 cup	1
Full fat: 1 cup	5	White: 1 cup	½

FRUIT

Apples, eating or cooking	0	Fig	0
Apricots	0	Grapefruit	0
Avocados, California:		Grapes	0
½ average size	6½	Lemons	0
Avocados, California, cubed:		Lime	0
1 cup	9	Mangoes	0
Avocados, California, purée:		Muskmelons, cantaloupe	0
1 cup	14	Nectarine	0
Avocados, Florida:		Orange	0
½ average size	6	Papaya	0
Avocados, Florida, cubed:		Peach	0
1 cup	6	Pear	0
Avocados, Florida, purée:		Pineapple	0
1 cup	9	Plums	0
Banana	0	Raspberries	0
Blackberries	0	Rhubarb	0
Blueberries	0	Strawberries	0
Cherries	0	Tangerines	0
Cranberries	0	Watermelon	0

			Fat Units
GELATIN, plain			0
Flavored, sweetened: ½ cup	3	Low calorie: ½ cup	1½

JUICES

Fresh fruit or vegetable	0

MACARONI	0

MARGARINE

Regular and soft: 1 tbsp	4	Diet: 1 tbsp	2
Whipped, soft: 1 tbsp	2	Imitation: 1 tbsp	2

MEAL

Almond meal, partially defatted:		Corn, white or yellow: 1 cup	1½
1 oz.	2	Crackermeal: 1 cup	½

MEAT, Fresh   3 oz.

Beef

Chuck:	
Boneless for stew:	
Lean with fat, cooked	7
Lean, cooked	3
Rib roast or chuck rib steak:	
Lean with fat, cooked	11
Lean, cooked	4
Arm and round bone roasts or steaks:	
Lean with fat, cooked	6
Lean, cooked	2
Flank steak:	
100% lean, cooked	1½
Ground beef:	
Regular (21% fat), raw	6
Lean (10% fat), raw	3
Rib roast, choice grade:	
Lean with fat, cooked	11½
Lean, cooked	4
Rump roast, choice grade:	
Lean with fat, cooked	8
Lean, cooked	3
Steaks:	
Club, choice grade:	
Lean with fat, cooked	12
Lean, cooked	4
Porterhouse, choice grade:	
Lean with fat, cooked	12
Lean, cooked	3
Sirloin, choice grade:	
Lean with fat, broiled	9½
Lean, broiled	3
Beef fat, cooked	24
Brains, beef and calf, raw	3

	Fat Units
Heart:	
Beef, lean, cooked	1½
Beef, lean with visible fat, cooked	9
Calf, cooked	3
Kidneys, beef and lamb, raw	1½
Liver:	
Beef, raw	1½
Calf, raw	1½
Sweetbreads, calf, raw	1½
Tongue:	
Beef, medium fat, raw	4½
Calf, raw	1½

Lamb

	Fat Units
Kidneys, raw	1½
Leg:	
Lean with fat, roasted	5½
Lean, cooked	2
Loin chops:	
Lean with fat, cooked	9½
1 chop (3 per lb.)	
Lean, cooked	2
1 chop (3 per lb.)	
Rib chops:	
Lean with fat, cooked	11
1 chop (3 per lb.)	
Lean, cooked	2
1 chop (3 per lb.)	
Shoulder:	
Lean with fat, cooked	8
Lean, cooked	3

Pork

	Fat Units
Ham:	
Lean with fat, cooked	9
Lean, cooked	3
Loin and loin chops:	
Lean with fat, cooked	8½
Lean, cooked	4½
Boston butt:	
Lean with fat, cooked	8½
Lean, roasted	4½
Picnic:	
Lean with fat, cooked	9
Lean, cooked	3
Spareribs, lean with fat, cooked	12

Veal

	Fat Units
Chuck cuts and boneless veal for stew, lean with fat, cooked	4
Loin, lean with fat, cooked	4
Rib roast, lean with fat, roasted	5
Round with rump (roasts and leg cutlets), lean with fat, cooked	3½

Fat Units

Other Meats

Rabbit, domesticated, stewed	3
Venison, lean meat only, raw	1½

MILK   1 cup unless noted

Milk, whole	3	Evaporated whole milk	6½
Lowfat milk (2% fat)	1½	Evaporated skim milk	0
Lowfat milk (1% fat)	1	Dried whole milk	12
Skim milk	0	Nonfat dry milk, regular and	
Chocolate milk	3	instant	½
Lowfat chocolate (2% fat)	2	Buttermilk, cultured	1
Lowfat chocolate (1% fat)	1		
Sweetened condensed whole milk	9½		

NOODLES   0

NUTS AND SEEDS   Nuts: 1 oz. = ¼ cup

Almonds:	
Chopped: 1 tbsp	1½
Slivered: 1 cup	22
Whole: 1 cup	27
Roasted in oil: 1 oz.	6
Dry roasted: 1 oz.	5½
Brazil nuts, shelled: 1 oz. or 6–8 kernels	6½
Cashew nuts:	
Roasted in oil: 1 oz.	5
Dry roasted: 1 oz.	4½
Chestnuts, fresh, shelled: 1 cup	1
Filberts, shelled, whole: 1 cup	29½
Peanuts:	
Roasted (Spanish and Virginia): 1 oz.	5½
Dry roasted: 1 oz.	5
Pecans:	
Chopped or pieces: 1 cup	29½
Chopped or pieces: 1 tbsp	2
Halves: 10 large	2½
Halves, roasted: 1 oz.	6½
Pine nuts, Pignolias, shelled: 1 oz.	4½
Pistachio nuts: 1 oz.	6
Walnuts:	
Black, shelled, chopped or broken kernels:	
1 cup	26
1 tbsp	1½
Persian or English, shelled, halves: 1 cup	22½
Persian or English, chopped: 1 tbsp	2
Persian or English: 10 large nuts	11
Seeds: 1 oz.	
Pumpkin	4½
Sesame	5½
Squash	4½
Sunflower	5

	Fat Units
OILS 1 tbsp	
Corn, cottonseed, peanut, olive, safflower, soybean, sunflower	5

OLIVES, green and ripe 3 olives	½

PEANUT BUTTER 1 tbsp	3

POPCORN

Popped, plain: 1 cup	0	Popped, with oil: 1 cup	½

POULTRY, Fresh

Chicken, broiled: ½ of 1¾-lb. broiler	2½
Chicken, fried, parts from 2½-lb. fryer:	
Back	3
Breast without ribs: ½ breast	2
Drumstick	1½
Neck	2½
Rib section: ½ section	½
Thigh	2
Wing	1½
Chicken, roasted:	
Light meat without skin: 3½ oz.	1½
Light meat without skin, chopped or diced: 1 cup	2½
Dark meat without skin: 3½ oz. (average drumstick)	2½
Dark meat without skin, chopped or diced: 1 cup	3
Chicken, stewed (hens and cocks):	
Meat and skin: 3½ oz.	8
Light meat without skin: 3½ oz.	1½
Dark meat without skin: 3½ oz.	3½
Chicken livers, raw: 3½ oz.	1½
Chicken livers, simmered: 3½ oz.	1½
Duck, domesticated, raw, meat only: 3½ oz.	3
Duck, wild, raw, meat only: 3½ oz.	2
Goose, domesticated, roasted:	
Meat only: 3½ oz.	3½
Meat and skin: 3½ oz.	13½
Turkey:	
Light meat without skin, roasted: 3½ oz.	1½
Dark meat without skin, roasted: 3½ oz.	3
Skin only, roasted: 3½ oz.	15
Giblets, simmered: 3½ oz.	5½

PRETZELS 1 oz.	½

RICE

Brown: 1 cup, cooked	0	White: 1 cup, cooked	0

ROLLS AND BUNS 1 oz.	½

SHELLFISH, Fresh   3 oz.

Abalone	½	Mussel	½
Clam	½	Oyster, Eastern and Pacific	½

Fat Units

Crab, blue, cooked	½	Periwinkle	1
Crab, soft shell	½	Scallop	½
Crab, Dungeness, meat	½	Shrimp	½
Crab, Alaska King, cooked,		Squid	½
legs and claws	½	Snail, pond	1
Lobster, Caribbean	½	Octopus	½
Lobster, rock, tail meat	½		

SHORTENING

Lard: 1 tbsp	4	Vegetable: 1 tbsp	4

SPAGHETTI   0

TORTILLA

Corn: 1 oz. (about 2 6½"-		Flour: 1 oz.	½
diameter tortillas)	½		

VEGETABLES, Fresh and Dried

Artichokes	0	Kale	0
Asparagus	0	Lentils	0
Bamboo shoots, raw	0	Lettuce	0
Barley, pearled, light:		Mushrooms	0
1 cup cooked	1	Mustard greens	0
Beans:		Okra	0
Great Northern, cooked,		Onions	0
drained	½	Parsnips	0
Lima (green)	½	Peas, green	0
Lima, mature	½	Peppers, green	0
Pea (navy)	½	Potatoes, baked or boiled	0
Red, kidney	½	Potato, French fried: 10 strips,	
Mung, sprouted seeds, raw	0	2-3½" long	2½
Snap, green, cooked	0	Potatoes, fried from raw: 1 cup	8½
Snap, yellow or wax, cooked	0	Potatoes, mashed with milk and	
Beets	0	butter or margarine: 1 cup	3
Beet greens	0	Pumpkin	0
Broccoli	0	Radishes	0
Cabbage	0	Rutabagas	0
Carrots	0	Soybeans, mature seeds, dry,	
Cauliflower	0	cooked: 1 cup	3½
Celery	0	Soybeans, sprouted seeds, raw:	
Chard, Swiss	0	1 cup	½
Chick peas or garbanzos:		Soybean curd (tofu): 1 piece	
1 cup cooked	½	2½ x2¾ x1"	2
Chives	0	Spinach	0
Collards	0	Squash	0
Corn, sweet, white and yellow,		Sweet potato	0
cooked	0	Tomatoes	0
Cucumbers	0	Turnips	0
Dandelion greens	0	Turnip greens	0
Eggplant	0	Watercress, raw, whole: 1 cup	0

TAPIOCA   0

			Fat Units
TEA			0
YEAST			0
YOGURT			
Regular: 1 cup	1½	Low fat: 1 cup	½

BRAND NAME FOODS

BISCUITS

	Fat Units
Refrigerator: 1 biscuit	
Ballard Oven Ready	½
1869 Brand	2
Hungry Jack Butter Tastin'	1½
Hungry Jack Flaky	1½
Pillsbury Country Style	½
Pillsbury Prize	1
Baking powder/1869 Brand	2
Baking powder, prebaked/1869 Brand	2
Baking powder/Tenderflake Dinner	1
Buttermilk:	
1869 Brand	2
1869 Brand, prebaked	2
Hungry Jack Extra Rich	1
Hungry Jack Flaky	½
Hungry Jack Fluffy	2
Pillsbury	½
Pillsbury Big Country	1
Pillsbury Extra Lights	½
Tenderflake Dinner	½
Cornbread/Pillsbury	1½

BREAD MIXES (prepared)

	Fat Units
Applesauce Spice: 1 loaf/Pillsbury	17
Apricot Nut: 1 loaf/Pillsbury	11½
Banana: 1 loaf/Pillsbury	17
Blueberry Nut: 1 loaf/Pillsbury	11½
Cherry Nut: 1 loaf/Pillsbury	17
Corn: 1 pkg/Aunt Jemima Easy Mix	15
Corn: 1 pkg/Pillsbury	11½
Cranberry: 1 loaf/Pillsbury	17
Date: 1 loaf/Pillsbury	11½
Nut: 1 loaf/Pillsbury	22½
Oatmeal Raisin: 1 loaf/Pillsbury	17

CAKES

	Fat Units
Frozen Cakes: 1 whole cake unless noted	
Banana/Pepperidge Farm	17
Banana/Sara Lee	19½
Black Forest/Sara Lee	26
Boston Creme/Pepperidge Farm	14
Cheesecake:	
Small/Sara Lee	17

	Fat Units
Mrs. Smith's	19
Chocolate:	
Pepperidge Farm	18½
Sara Lee	25
Double layer/Sara Lee	35
Bavarian/Sara Lee	57
Fudge/Pepperidge Farm	32
Fudge/Pepperidge Farm Half Cakes	16
German/Pepperidge Farm	21
German/Sara Lee	32
Coconut/Pepperidge Farm	32
Coconut/Pepperidge Farm Half Cake	16
Coffee cake:	
Almond/Sara Lee	25
Pecan, large/Sara Lee	26
Pecan, small/Sara Lee	15
Streusel, cinnamon/Sara Lee	24½
Streusel, large butter/Sara Lee	30
Coffee Ring, almond/Sara Lee	23½
Coffee Ring, blueberry/Sara Lee	17½
Coffee Ring, maple crunch/Sara Lee	27
Coffee Ring, raspberry/Sara Lee	20
Crumbcake:	
Blueberry/Sara Lee	2
Blueberry/Stouffer	3
Chocolate Chip/Stouffer	4
French/Sara Lee	2½
French/Stouffer	3
Cupcake:	
Chocolate/Sara Lee	3
Chocolate, double/Sara Lee	3
Cream-filled/Stouffer	4
Yellow/Sara Lee	2½
Yellow/Stouffer	3
Devil's Food/Pepperidge Farm	28
Devil's Food/Sara Lee	28
Golden/Pepperidge Farm Half Cakes	16
Golden/Sara Lee	22
Golden Layer/Pepperidge Farm	32
Lemon Bavarian/Sara Lee	54½
Lemon Coconut/Pepperidge Farm	15½
Mandarin Orange layer/Sara Lee	29½
Pound Cake:	
Sara Lee	23½
Apple Nut/Pepperidge Farm Old Fashioned	17½
Banana Nut/Sara Lee	20
Butter/Pepperidge Farm Old Fashioned	24½
Carrot/Pepperidge Farm Old Fashioned	32
Chocolate/Pepperidge Farm Old Fashioned	24½
Chocolate/Sara Lee	28
Chocolate Swirl/Sara Lee	20
Family Size/Sara Lee	36

	Fat Units
Home Style/Sara Lee	21
Raisin/Sara Lee	20½
Orange Cake/Sara Lee	22½
Cherry Shortcake/Mrs. Smith's	38
Strawberry Shortcake/Sara Lee	25½
Strawberry Shortcake/Mrs. Smith's	38
Strawberry 'n Cream layer/Sara Lee	31½
Vanilla/Pepperidge Farm	28
Walnut layer/Sara Lee	36½
Mixes: Prepared according to package directions, 1 whole cake	
Angel Food/various brands	22
Apple Raisin/Duncan Hines	21
Apple Raisin, Spicy/Duncan Hines Moist and Easy	12½
Applesauce Raisin/Betty Crocker Snackin' Cake	19
Banana/Betty Crocker	55
Banana/Duncan Hines Supreme	21
Banana/Pillsbury Plus	51
Banana Nut/Duncan Hines Moist and Easy	22
Banana Walnut/Betty Crocker Snackin' Cake	22
Bundt cake:	
Chocolate Macaroon/Pillsbury	59½
Fudge Nut Crown/Pillsbury	51
Lemon Blueberry/Pillsbury	46½
Marble/Pillsbury	51
Pound/Pillsbury	51
Triple Fudge/Pillsbury	55
Butter and Butter Fudge/Duncan Hines	55
Butter/Pillsbury Plus	42½
Butter Brickle/Betty Crocker	51
Butter Pecan/Betty Crocker	55
Cheesecake/Pillsbury No Bake	141
Cheesecake/Jell-O	31
Cheesecake/Royal	8½
Cherry/Duncan Hines	21
Cherry Chip/Betty Crocker	21
Chocolate/Betty Crocker Pudding Cake	10½
Chocolate/Duncan Hines	25½
Chocolate Almond/Betty Crocker Snackin' Cake	25½
Chocolate Chip/Betty Crocker Snackin' Cake	25½
Chocolate Chip/Duncan Hines	19
Chocolate Chip, double/Duncan Hines	16
Chocolate, dark/Pillsbury Plus	51
Chocolate Fudge/Betty Crocker Snackin' Cake	25½
Chocolate Fudge/Betty Crocker	59½
Chocolate, German/Betty Crocker	55
Chocolate, German/Pillsbury	51
Chocolate, milk/Betty Crocker	51
Chocolate, sour cream/Betty Crocker	59½
Chocolate, sour cream/Duncan Hines	25½
Chocolate, Swiss/Duncan Hines	25½
Chocolate, with chocolate frosting/Betty Crocker Stir n' Frost	23½
Coconut Pecan/Betty Crocker Snackin' Cake	28½

	Fat Units
Cupcakes/Flako	2
Date Nut/Betty Crocker Snackin' Cake	25½
Devil's Food/Betty Crocker	55
Devil's Food/Duncan Hines	25½
Devil's Food/Pillsbury	51
Fudge Marble/Duncan Hines	21
Fudge Marble/Pillsbury	51
Gingerbread/Betty Crocker	19
Gingerbread: 3" sq/Pillsbury	1½
Lemon/Betty Crocker Pudding Cake	10½
Lemon, with lemon frosting/Betty Crocker Stir n' Frost	17
Lemon/Betty Crocker	55
Lemon/Duncan Hines	21
Lemon/Pillsbury	51
Lemon Chiffon/Betty Crocker	17
Marble/Betty Crocker	55
Orange/Betty Crocker	55
Orange/Duncan Hines	21
Pineapple/Duncan Hines	21
Pineapple Upside-Down, with topping/Betty Crocker	32
Pound/Betty Crocker	34
Spice/Betty Crocker	59½
Spice/Duncan Hines	21
Spice, with vanilla frosting/Betty Crocker Stir n' Frost	17
Spice Raisin/Betty Crocker Snackin' Cake	19
Strawberry/Betty Crocker	55
Strawberry/Duncan Hines	21
Strawberry/Pillsbury	51
Streusel cake:	
Cinnamon/Pillsbury	59½
Devil's Food/Pillsbury	55
Fudge Marble/Pillsbury	59½
German Chocolate/Pillsbury	55
Lemon/Pillsbury	63½
Yellow/Betty Crocker	55
Yellow/Betty Crocker Butter Recipe	42½
Yellow/Duncan Hines	21
Yellow, with chocolate frosting/Betty Crocker Stir n' Frost	17
Yellow/Pillsbury	51
White/Betty Crocker	25½
White/Duncan Hines	21
White/Pillsbury	42½
White, sour cream/Betty Crocker	25½
Coffee Cakes: 1 whole cake	
Apple Cinnamon, mix, prepared/Pillsbury	20
Butter Pecan, mix, prepared/Pillsbury	42½
Cinnamon Streusel, mix, prepared/Pillsbury	22½
Coffee Cake, mix, prepared/Aunt Jemima Easy Mix	14
Sour Cream, mix, prepared/Pillsbury	34

	Fat Units
CAKES, Snack	
Big Wheels: 1 cake/Hostess	3½
Brownie, large: 1 brownie/Hostess	3½
Choco-Diles: 1 cake/Hostess	4
Creamies, chocolate or spice: 1 pkg/Tastykake	3½
Crumb Cake: 1 cake/Hostess	1½
Cupcakes:	
Butter-cream filled: 1 pkg/Tastykake	3
Chocolate: 1 cake/Hostess	2
Chocolate: 1 pkg/Tastykake	2
Ding Dongs: 1 cake/Hostess	3½
Donuts:	
Hostess, plain: 1 donut	2½
Hostess Crunch: 1 donut	1½
Hostess Enrobed: 1 donut	3
Cinnamon or powdered: 1 donut/Hostess	2
Ho Hos: 1 cake/Hostess	2
Juniors, chocolate: 1 pkg/Tastykake	4½
Juniors, coconut: 1 pkg/Tastykake	4
Juniors, koffee kake: 1 pkg/Tastykake	5½
Juniors, lemon: 1 pkg/Tastykake	2½
Koffee Kake, cream-filled: 1 pkg/Tastykake	4
Krimpets, butterscotch: 1 pkg/Tastykake	2
Krimpets, jelly: 1 pkg/Tastykake	1
Krimpies, chocolate: 1 pkg/Tastykake	3
Krimpies, vanilla: 1 pkg/Tastykake	3
Macaroon, fudge: 1 cake/Hostess	3
Oatmeal Cake, creme-filled: 2 oz./Frito-Lay's	4
Oatmeal Raisin: 1 pkg/Tastykake Bars	3½
Orange Treats: 1 pkg/Tastykake	2½
Sno Balls: 1 cake/Hostess	1½
Suzy Q: 1 cake/Hostess	3
Tandy Takes, peanut butter: 1 pkg/Tastykake	4
Tandy Takes, chocolate: 1 pkg/Tastykake	3½
Tasty Klairs, chocolate: 1 pkg/Tastykake	8½
Teens, chocolate: 1 pkg/Tastykake	2
Tempty, chocolate cream: 1 pkg/Tastykake	1½
Tempty, lemon: 1 pkg/Tastykake	3
Tiger Tails: 1 cake/Hostess	4½
Twinkies: 1 cake/Hostess	1½
Twinkies, devil's food: 1 cake/Hostess	2
CANDY	
Chocolate and chocolate covered bars:	
Hershey's, plain and with almonds: 1 oz.	3½
Nestlé, plain and with almonds: 1 oz.	3
Baby Ruth: 1 bar	4
Butterfinger: 1 bar	3½
Choco'Lite: 1 oz./Nestlé	3

	Fat Units
Choc-O-Roon: 2 oz./Frito Lay's	5½
Crunch: 1 oz./Nestlé	3
Kit Kat: 1.1 oz./Hershey's	3
Krackel: 1 oz./Hershey's	3
Mr. Goodbar: 1.3 oz.	4½
$100,000: 1 oz./Nestlé	2
Rally: 1.5 oz./Hershey's	4
Reggie: 1 bar	6
Special Dark Bar/Hershey's: 1.2 oz.	3½
Chocolate and chocolate bits:	
Hershey-ets: 1.1 oz.	2
Kisses: 1 oz./Hershey's	3
Rolo: 1 piece/Hershey's	½
Peanut Candy, canned: 1 oz./Planters Old Fashioned	3
Peanut Butter Bar: 1¾ oz./Frito-Lay's	6
Peanut Butter Cup: 1 piece/Reese's	2

CEREALS

Dry Ready-to-Serve: Measurements vary according to what companies consider appropriate 1-serving sizes. The servings generally are 1 ounce in weight. Fat units have been adjusted to reflect the higher sugar content of some cereals.

All-Bran: ⅓ cup/Kellogg's	½
Alpha-Bits: 1 cup/Post	½
Apple Jacks: 1 cup/Kellogg's	½
Boo Berry: 1 cup/General Mills	½
Bran, plain	½
Bran Buds: ⅓ cup/Kellogg's	½
Bran Chex: ⅔ cup/Ralston Purina	½
Bran Flakes 40%: ⅔ cup/Kellogg's	½
Bran Flakes: ⅔ cup/Post 40%	½
Buc Wheats: ¾ cup/General Mills	½
C.W. Post: ½ cup	1½
C.W. Post, with raisins: ½ cup	1½
Cap'n Crunch: ¾ cup	1
Cap'n Crunch's Crunchberries: ¾ cup	1
Cap'n Crunch's Peanut Butter: ¾ cup	1
Cheerios: 1¼ cups/General Mills	½
Chocolate Crazy Cow: 1 cup/General Mills	½
Cocoa Krispies: ¾ cup/Kellogg's	½
Cocoa Pebbles: ⅞ cup/Post	1
Cocoa Puffs: 1 cup/General Mills	½
Concentrate: ⅓ cup/Kellogg's	½
Cookie Crisp: 1 cup/Ralston Purina	½
Corn Chex: 1 cup/Ralston Purina	½
Corn Flakes: 1 cup/General Mills Country	½
Corn Flakes: 1 cup/Kellogg's	½
Corn Flakes: 1¼ cups/Post Toasties	½
Corn Flakes: 1 cup/Ralston Purina	½
Corn Flakes, sugar coated: ⅔ cup/Kellogg's Frosted	1½
Corn Total: 1 cup/General Mills	½

	Fat Units
Corny-Snaps: 1 cup/Kellogg's	1
Count Chocula: 1 cup/General Mills	½
Country Morning: ⅓ cup/Kellogg's	2
Country Morning, with raisins and dates: ⅓ cup/Kellogg's	2
Cracklin' Bran: ⅓ cup/Kellogg's	1½
Crispy Rice: 1 cup/Ralston Purina	½
Franken Berry: 1 cup/General Mills	½
Froot Loops: 1 cup/Kellogg's	½
Frosty O's: 1 cup/General Mills	½
Fruit Brute: 1 cup/General Mills	½
Fruity Pebbles: ⅞ cup/Post	1
Golden Grahams: 1 cup/General Mills	½
Granola: 1 oz./Nature Valley	2
Granola, with cinnamon and raisins: 1 oz./Nature Valley	2
Granola, with coconut and honey: 1 oz./Nature Valley	2
Granola, with fruit and nuts: 1 oz./Nature Valley	1½
Grape Nuts: ¼ cup/Post	½
Grape Nut Flakes: ⅞ cup/Post	½
Honeycomb: 1⅓ cups/Post	½
Kaboom: 1 cup/General Mills	½
King Vitaman: ¾ cup/Quaker	1
Kix: 1½ cups/General Mills	½
Life: ⅔ cup/Quaker	½
Lucky Charms: 1 cup/General Mills	½
Mini-Wheats: about 5 biscuits/Kellogg's	½
Oat Flakes, fortified: ⅔ cup/Post	½
Pep: ¾ cup/Kellogg's	½
Product 19: ¾ cup/Kellogg's	½
Quaker 100% Natural: ¼ cup	2
Quaker 100% Natural, with apples and cinnamon: ¼ cup	2
Quaker 100% Natural, with raisins and dates: ¼ cup	2
Quisp: 1⅙ cups	1
Raisin Bran: ¾ cup/Kellogg's	½
Raisin Bran: ½ cup/Post	½
Raisin Bran: ½ cup/Ralston Purina	½
Rice: 1 cup/Safeway Crispy Rice	½
Rice, frosted: 1 cup/Kellogg's	½
Rice Krinkles, frosted: ⅞ cup/Post	½
Rice, puffed: ½ oz./Malt-O-Meal	½
Rice, puffed: 1 cup/Quaker	½
Rice Chex, 1⅛ cups/Ralston Purina	½
Rice Krispies: 1 cup/Kellogg's	½
Special K: 1¼ cups/Kellogg's	½
Strawberry Crazy Cow: 1 cup/General Mills	½
Sugar Corn Pops: 1 cup/Kellogg's	½
Sugar Frosted Flakes: ¾ cup/Ralston Purina	1
Sugar Smacks: ¾ cup/Kellogg's	1
Toasty O's: 1 oz.	½
Total: 1 cup/General Mills	½
Trix: 1 cup/General Mills	½
Wheat, puffed: ½ oz./Malt-O-Meal	½
Wheat, puffed: 1 cup/Quaker	½

	Fat Units
Wheat, shredded: 1 biscuit/Quaker	½
Wheat Chex: ⅔ cup/Ralston Purina	½
Super Sugar Crisp: ⅞ cup/Post	½
Wheaties: 1 cup/General Mills	½
To Be Cooked: Measurements vary	
Barley, pearled: ¼ cup uncooked (1 cup cooked)/Quaker Scotch Brand	½
Farina: 1 cup cooked/various brands	½
Grits: ¼ cup uncooked/various brands	½
Grits, with artificial cheese flavor: 1 packet/Quaker Instant Grits Product	½
Grits, with imitation bacon or ham bits: 1 packet/Quaker Instant Grits Product	½
Malt-O-Meal Chocolate: 1 oz. uncooked (about ¾ cup cooked)	½
Malt-O-Meal Quick: 1 oz. uncooked (about ¾ cup cooked)	½
Oats and Oatmeal, regular and instant unsweetened: 1 serving/ about ¾ cup cooked various brands	½
Oats, Quaker Instant: 1 packet	
with apples and cinnamon	1½
with bran and raisins	2
with cinnamon and spice	2½
with maple and brown sugar	2
with raisins and spice	2
Ralston: 1 oz. (uncooked)/Ralston Purina	½
Ralston: 1 oz. (uncooked)/Ralston Purina Instant	½
Whole Wheat: ⅓ cup uncooked (⅔ cup cooked)/Quaker Pettijohns	½

CHINESE FOOD

Apple Cinnamon Roll, frozen: 1 roll/La Choy	½
Bamboo Shoots, canned: 8½ oz. can/Chun King	0
Bean Sprouts, canned: 16 oz. can/Chun King	0
Bean Sprouts, canned: 1 cup/La Choy	0
Chop Suey, beef, frozen: 7 oz./Banquet Cookin' Bag	½
Chop Suey, vegetables, canned: 1 cup/La Choy	0
Chow mein, canned:	
Beef: 1 cup/La Choy	1
Chicken: 1 cup/La Choy	1
Meatless: 1 cup/La Choy	½
Mushroom: 1 cup/La Choy	1
Pepper Oriental: 1 cup/La Choy	½
Pepper Oriental: 1 cup/La Choy Bi-Pack	½
Pork: 1 cup/La Choy Bi-Pack	2
Shrimp: 1 cup/La Choy	½
Vegetables: 16 oz. can/Chun King	0
Chow mein, frozen:	
Beef, La Choy	½
Chicken: 7 oz./Banquet Cookin' Bag	½
Chicken: 1 cup/La Choy	1½
Chicken, without noodles: 9 oz./Green Giant Boil-in-Bag	½
Shrimp: 1 cup/La Choy	½
Egg Rolls, chicken, frozen: 1 roll/La Choy	½
Egg Rolls, lobster, frozen: 1 roll/La Choy	½
Fried Rice, chicken, canned: 1 cup/La Choy	1½

	Fat Units
Fried Rice, Chinese style, canned: 1 cup/La Choy	1½
Fried Rice & Pork, frozen: 1 cup/La Choy	2
Noodles, chow mein, canned: 1 cup/La Choy	6
Noodles, ramen-beef, canned: 1 cup/La Choy	2½
Noodles, ramen-chicken, canned: 1 cup/La Choy	2½
Noodles, ramen-oriental, canned: 1 cup/La Choy	3
Noodles, rice, canned: 1 cup/La Choy	3½
Pea Pods, frozen: 1 pkg/La Choy	0
Pepper Oriental, frozen: 1 cup/La Choy	½
Sweet & Sour Pork, frozen: 1 cup/La Choy	2
Vegetables, mixed Chinese, canned: 1 cup/La Choy	0
Water Chestnuts, canned: 8½ oz./Chun King	0
Won Ton, frozen: 1 cup/La Choy	½

CHIPS, CRISPS, AND SIMILAR SNACKS

	Fat Units
Cheddar Bitz: 1 oz./Frito-Lay's	1½
Cheez Balls: 1 oz./Planters	3½
Chee Tos: 1 oz./Frito-Lay's	3½
Corn chips: 1 oz.:	
Fritos	3½
Planters	4
Barbecue flavored: 1 oz./Fritos	3½
Corn Nuggets, toasted: 1⅜ oz./Frito-Lay's	2
Funyuns: 1 oz.	2
Munchos: 1 oz./Frito-Lay's	3½
Potato chips: 1 oz.:	
Frito-Lay's	4
Planters Stackable	3
Pringles	3½
Pringle's Country Style	4
Potato Sticks, canned: 1½ oz./O&C	5½
Rinds, fried, pork: 1 oz./Baken-Ets	2½
Sesame Nut Mix: 1 oz./Planters	4½
Snack Sticks: 1 oz./Pepperidge Farm	1½
Tortilla Chips: 1 oz./Doritos	2½
Tortilla Chips: 1 oz./Planters Nacho and Taco	2½
Wheat Chips, imitation bacon flavored: 1 oz./Bakon-Snacks	3

CHOCOLATE AND CHIPS

For Baking

	Fat Units
Chips:	
Butterscotch flavored: 1 oz./Nestlé Morsels	2½
Chocolate: ¼ cup/Hershey's	5
Chocolate: 1 oz./Nestlé Morsels	3
Chocolate, flavor: 1 oz. (2½ tbsp)/Baker's	2½
Chocolate, semi-sweet: 1.5 oz./Hershey's	4
Peanut butter flavored: 1 oz./Reese's	3
Choco-bake 1 oz./Nestlé	5
Chocolate, solid: 1 oz./Hershey's	5½
Chocolate, unswt: 1 oz./Baker's	5

	Fat Units
Chocolate, solid, semi-sweet or German's: 1 oz./Baker's	3
Cocoa: 1 oz.	1½
Cocoa mix: 1 oz.	½

CONDIMENTS

A.1 Sauce: 1 tbsp	0
Catsup/various brands	0
Hot Sauce: 1 tsp/Frank's	0
Mustard, prepared: 1 tsp/various brands	0
Seafood, cocktail: ¼ cup/Del Monte	½
Seafood, cocktail: 2 oz./Pfeiffer	1½
Soy Sauce: 1 tbsp/various brands	0
Taco Sauce: 1 tbsp/Ortega	0
Tartar Sauce: 1 tbsp/Best Foods	3
Tartar Sauce: 1 tbsp/Hellmann's	3
Tartar Sauce: 1 tbsp/Seven Seas	3
Vinegar/various brands	0
Worcestershire: 1 tbsp/French's	0

COOKIES   1 piece as pkg unless noted

Adelaide: Pepperidge Farm	1
Angel Puffs: Stella D'Oro Dietetic	½
Angelica Goodies: Stella D'Oro	1½
Anginetti: Stella D'Oro	½
Animal crackers: 2 cookies/Sunshine	½
Animal crackers, iced: Sunshine	½
Animal crackers, 2 cookies/Barnum's Animals: Nabisco	½
Anisette Sponge: Stella D'Oro	½
Anisette Toast: Stella D'Oro	½
Applesauce: Sunshine	1½
Arrowroot: Sunshine	½
Assortment: Stella D'Oro	½
Aunt Sally, iced: Sunshine	1
Big Treat: Sunshine	2
Biscos/Nabisco	½
Bordeaux: Pepperidge Farm	½
Breakfast Treats: Stella D'Oro	1½
Brown Sugar: Pepperidge Farm	1
Brussels: Pepperidge Farm	1
Butter Flavored/Nabisco	½
Butter Flavored/Sunshine	½
Cameo Creme Sandwich/Nabisco	1
Capri: Pepperidge Farm	2
Chessman: Pepperidge Farm	½
Chinese Dessert Cookies: Stella D'Oro	3
Chip-A-Roos: Sunshine	1
Chocolate Brownie: Pepperidge Farm	1½
Chocolate Chip: Pepperidge Farm	½
Chocolate Chip Coconut: Sunshine	1½
Chocolate Fudge Sandwich: Sunshine	1½

	Fat Units
Cinnamon Sugar: Pepperidge Farm	1
Cinnamon Toast: 2 cookies/Sunshine	½
Coconut Bar/Sunshine	1
Coconut Cookies/Stella D'Oro Dietetic	1
Coconut Macaroons/Nabisco	1½
Como Delight/Stella D'Oro	2½
Cream Lunch/Sunshine	½
Crescents, almond-flavored/Nabisco	½
Cup Custard, chocolate/Sunshine	1
Cup Custard, vanilla/Sunshine	1
Date-Nut Granola: Pepperidge Farm	1
Dixie Vanilla: Sunshine	½
Egg Biscuits: Stella D'Oro	½
Egg Biscuits: Stella D'Oro Roman	2
Egg Biscuits, sugared: Stella D'Oro	½
Egg Jumbo: Stella D'Oro	½
Fig Bars: Sunshine	½
Fig Pastry: Stella D'Oro Dietetic	1½
Fudge Chip/Pepperidge Farm	1
Ginger Snaps/Nabisco	½
Ginger Snaps/Sunshine	½
Gingerman/Pepperidge Farm	½
Golden Bars/Stella D'Oro	1½
Golden Fruit/Sunshine	½
Graham Crackers: 1 piece/Nabisco Honey Maid	½
Graham Crackers/Sunshine Sweet-Tooth	1
Honey Grahams: 1 entire piece/Sunshine	?
Hydrox: Sunshine	1
Irish Oatmeal: Pepperidge Farm	1
Kichel, 3 cookies, Stella D'Oro Dietetic	½
Lady Joan/Sunshine	1
LaLanne/Sunshine	½
Lemon/Sunshine	1½
Lemon Coolers/Sunshine	½
Lemon Nut Crunch/Pepperidge Farm	1
Lido/Pepperidge Farm	2
Love Cookies/Stella D'Oro Dietetic	2
Mallopuffs/Sunshine	½
Margherite/Stella D'Oro	1
Milano/Pepperidge Farm	1½
Molasses Crisps/Pepperidge Farm	½
Molasses and Spice/Sunshine	½
Nassau/Pepperidge Farm	1½
'Nilla Wafers, 2 cookies, Nabisco	½
Nutter Butter/Nabisco	1
Oatmeal:	
Sunshine	1
Almond/Pepperidge Farm	1
Iced/Sunshine	1
Marmalade/Pepperidge Farm	1
Peanut Butter/Sunshine	1½
Raisin/Nabisco	1
Raisin/Pepperidge Farm	1

	Fat Units
Orbit Creme Sandwich/Sunshine	1
Oreo/Nabisco	½
Orleans/Pepperidge Farm	½
Peanut/Pepperidge Farm	1
Peanut Butter Wafers/Sunshine	½
Peanut Creme Patties/Nabisco	½
Pirouette/Pepperidge Farm	1
Pirouette, chocolate laced/Pepperidge Farm	1
Pfeffernusse/Stella D'Oro Spice Drops	½
Raisin Bran/Pepperidge Farm	1
Raisin Fruit Biscuit/Nabisco	½
Royal Nuggets/Stella D'Oro Dietetic	0
St. Mortiz/Pepperidge Farm	1
Sandwich:	
Assortment/Nabisco Pride	1
Creme, Swiss/Nabisco	1
Scotties/Sunshine	½
Sesame Cookies/Stella D'Oro Regina	1
Sesame Cookies/Stella D'Oro Regina Dietetic	1
Shortbread/Pepperidge Farm	1½
Shortbread, pecan/Nabisco	1½
Social Tea Biscuit, 3 cookies, Nabisco	½
Social Tea Sandwich/Nabisco	1
Sorrento Cookies/Stella D'Oro	1
Sprinkles/Sunshine	½
Sugar/Pepperidge Farm	1
Sugar/Sunshine	1½
Sugar Rings/Nabisco	1
Sunflower Raisin/Pepperidge Farm	1
Swiss Fudge/Stella D'Oro	1½
Tahiti/Pepperidge Farm	2
Taste of Vienna/Stella D'Oro	1½
Toy cookies, 2 cookies, Sunshine	½
Vanilla Snaps/Nabisco	½
Vienna Finger Sandwich/Sunshine	1
Wafers:	
Brown Edge/Nabisco	½
Spiced/Nabisco	½
Sugar/Biscos	½
Sugar/Sunshine	½
Sugar, lemon/Sunshine	½
Vanilla, 2 cookies, Sunshine	½
Yum Yums/Sunshine	1
Zanzibar/Pepperidge Farm	1
Zuzu Ginger Snaps, 2 cookies, Nabisco	½

CRACKERS 1 cracker unless noted

Cheez-Its, 6 crackers, Sunshine	½
Cheese-filled: 1½ oz./Frito-Lay's	3½
Fling Curls/Nabisco	½

	Fat Units
Goldfish: 1 oz./Pepperidge Farm	2½
Goldfish, pretzel: 1 oz./Pepperidge Farm	1
Goldfish, thins: 4 thins/Pepperidge Farm	1
Goldfish, thins, wheat: 4 thins/Pepperidge Farm	1½
Hi Ho/Sunshine	½
Kavli Flatbread: 1 wafer	½
Matzos: 1 sheet or 1 cracker/Manischewitz	½
Mixed Suites, green onion: 1 oz./Pepperidge Farm	2
Mixed Suites, pretzel-cheese: 1 oz./Pepperidge Farm	1
Mixed Suites, sesame-cheese: 1 oz./Pepperidge Farm	2½
Oyster, 12 crackers, Sunshine	½
Peanut butter: 1½ oz./Frito-Lay's	3½
Ritz: Nabisco	½
Ritz Cheese, 2 crackers, Nabisco	½
Saltines and soda crackers, 2 crackers, various brands	½
Shapies, cheese-flavored, 3 crackers, Nabisco	½
Sip 'N Chips, cheese-flavored, 3 crackers, Nabisco	½
Sociables, 3 crackers, Nabisco	½
Triangle Thins, 4 crackers, Nabisco	½
Triscuit/Nabisco	½
Twigs/Nabisco	½
Waverly Wafers/Nabisco	½
Wheat Thins, 4 crackers, Nabisco	½
Zwieback/Nabisco	½

CREAMERS, NONDAIRY

Dry:	
Carnation Coffee-Mate: 1 packet	½
Coffee Tone: 1 tsp	½
Cremora: 1 tsp	½
Liquid:	
Coffee Tone Freezer Pack: 1 tbsp	½
Rich's: 1 tbsp	½

CROUTONS

Pepperidge Farm: 1 oz.	2

DIET BARS 1 bar

Carnation Slender Bars	2½
Pillsbury Food Sticks	½
Pillsbury Figurines	3

DINNERS

Frozen Dinners: 1 dinner	
Beans and Beef Patties: 11 oz./Swanson "TV"	6
Beans and Franks: 10¾ oz./Morton	6
Beans and Franks: 11¼ oz./Swanson "TV"	7

	Fat Units
Beef:	
Banquet/11 oz.	4
La Choy	2½
Morton: 10 oz.	4
Swanson "TV": 11½ oz.	4
Swanson 3 Course/15 oz.	6
Beef, chopped: 11 oz./Banquet	9½
Beef, chopped: 11 oz./Morton	8
Beef, sirloin chopped: 10 oz./Swanson "TV"	9
Beef, sliced: 14 oz./Morton Country Table	7
Beef, sliced: 17 oz./Swanson Hungry-Man	6½
Chicken: La Choy	3
Chicken, boneless: 10 oz./Morton	2½
Chicken, boneless: 19 oz./Swanson Hungry-Man	10
Chicken, breast: 15 oz./Weight Watchers	2½
Chicken, croquette: 10¼ oz./Morton	6½
Chicken, fried:	
Banquet: 11 oz.	9
Morton: 11 oz.	5
Morton Country Table: 15 oz.	6½
Swanson "TV": 11½ oz.	10
Barbecue flavored: 11¼ oz./Swanson "TV"	9
Crispy fried: 10¾ oz./Swanson "TV"	12
Chicken and Dumplings: 12 oz./Banquet	3
Chicken with Dumplings: 11 oz./Morton	3½
Chicken and Noodles: 12 oz./Banquet	3½
Chicken with Noodles: 10¼ oz./Morton	2½
Chicken Oriental Style: 15 oz./Weight Watchers	2
Chop Suey, beef: 12 oz./Banquet	3
Chow Mein, chicken: 12 oz./Banquet	4½
Enchilada, beef: 12 oz./Banquet	6
Enchilada, beef: 15 oz./Swanson "TV"	8
Enchilada, cheese: 12 oz./Banquet	6
Fish: 8¾ oz./Banquet	5
Fish: 9 oz./Morton	3
Fish 'n' Chips: 10¼ oz./Swanson "TV"	7
Flounder: 16 oz./Weight Watchers	1
German Style: 11¾ oz./Swanson "TV"	6
Haddock: 8¾ oz./Banquet	6
Haddock: 16 oz./Weight Watchers	1
Ham: 10¼ oz./Swanson "TV"	4½
Ham: 10 oz./Banquet	4½
Ham: 10 oz./Morton	6
Hash, corned beef: 10 oz./Banquet	4½
Italian Style: 11 oz./Banquet	7½
Italian Style: 13 oz./Swanson "TV"	6
Macaroni and Beef: 12 oz./Banquet	5
Macaroni and Beef: 10 oz./Morton	2
Macaroni and Beef: 12 oz./Swanson "TV"	5½
Macaroni and Cheese: 12 oz./Banquet	3½
Macaroni and Cheese: 11 oz./Morton	3
Macaroni and Cheese: 12½ oz./Swanson "TV"	5

	Fat Units
Meat Loaf: 11 oz./Banquet	8½
Meat Loaf: 11 oz./Morton	5½
Meat Loaf: 15 oz./Morton Country Table	5½
Meat Loaf: 10¾ oz./Swanson "TV"	10
Meatballs: 11¾ oz./Swanson "TV"	8½
Mexican Style: 16 oz./Banquet	9
Mexican Style Combination: 12 oz./Banquet	7½
Mexican Style Combination: 16 oz./Swanson "TV"	9
Noodles and Chicken: 10¼ oz./Swanson "TV"	5½
Pepper Oriental/La Choy	2½
Perch, ocean: 8¾ oz./Banquet	6
Perch, ocean: 16 oz./Weight Watchers	4
Polynesian Style: 13 oz./Swanson "TV"	6
Pork, loin of: 11¼ oz./Swanson "TV"	8
Salisbury Steak:	
Banquet/11 oz.	8½
Morton/11 oz.	4½
Morton Country Table/15 oz.	5½
Swanson "TV"/11½ oz.	10
Swanson 3 course/16 oz.	8½
Shrimp/La Choy	2
Sole: 16 oz./Weight Watchers	1
Spaghetti and Meatballs: 11½ oz./Banquet	5½
Spaghetti and Meatballs: 11 oz./Morton	3
Spaghetti and Meatballs: 12½ oz./Swanson "TV"	5
Spaghetti and Meatballs: 18½ oz./Swanson Hungry-Man	9
Swiss Steak: 10 oz./Swanson "TV"	4½
Turbot: 16 oz./Weight Watchers	8
Turkey:	
Banquet/11 oz.	3½
Banquet Man-Pleaser/19 oz.	6½
Morton/11 oz.	5
Morton Country Table/15 oz.	6
Swanson "TV"/11½ oz.	4
Swanson 3 Course/16 oz.	7½
Breast: 16 oz./Weight Watchers	4
Veal Parmigiana: 11 oz./Banquet	6½
Veal Parmigiana: 10¼ oz./Morton	3
Veal Parmigiana: 12¼ oz./Swanson "TV"	9½
Western: 11 oz./Banquet	8½
Western Round-Up: 11¾ oz./Morton	8
Western Style: 11¾ oz./Swanson "TV"	8

DINNER MIXES

Hamburger Helper: ⅕ prepared dinner/Betty Crocker	5½
Tuna Helper: ⅕ prepared dinner/Betty Crocker	2½

EGG MIXES

Egg, imitation, frozen: ¼ cup/Morningstar Farms Scramblers	1
Egg, imitation, mix: ½ pkg/Eggstra	½
Egg, imitation, refrigerated: ¼ cup/No-fat Egg Beaters	0

	Fat Units
Egg mixes and seasonings	
Omelet, bacon, dry mix: 1 pkg/Durkee	½
Omelet, cheese, dry mix: 1 pkg/Durkee	2½
Omelet, Western: 1 pkg/Durkee (add water only)	2
Scrambled: 1 pkg/Durkee (add water only)	3½
Scrambled, with bacon, 1 pkg/Durkee (add water only)	4½

GRAVIES

	Fat Units
Au jus:	
Mix, prepared: ¼ cup/Durkee	0
Mix, prepared: ¼ cup/French's	0
Mix, prepared: ¼ cup/French's Pan Rich	½
Beef, canned: 2 oz./Franco-American	½
Brown:	
Mix, prepared: ¼ cup/Durkee	0
Mix, prepared: ¼ cup/French's	½
Mix, prepared: ¼ cup/French's Pan Rich	2
Mix, prepared: ¼ cup/Pillsbury	0
Mix, prepared: ¼ cup/Spatini Family Style	0
Mix, prepared: ¼ cup/Weight Watchers	0
With mushrooms, mix, prepared: ¼ cup/Durkee	0
With mushrooms, mix, prepared: ¼ cup/Weight Watchers	0
With onions, canned: 2 oz./Franco-American	½
With onions, mix, prepared: ¼ cup/Durkee	0
With onions, mix, prepared: ¼ cup/Weight Watchers	0
Chicken:	
Canned: 2 oz./Franco-American	1½
Mix, prepared: ¼ cup/Durkee	½
Mix, prepared: ¼ cup/Durkee Creamy	1
Mix, prepared: ¼ cup/French's	½
Mix, prepared: ¼ cup/French's Pan Rich	2
Mix, prepared: ¼ cup/Pillsbury	½
Mix, prepared: ¼ cup/Weight Watchers	0
Creamy, mix, with roasting bag: 1 pkg/Durkee Roastin' Bag	4
Chicken Giblet, canned: 2 oz./Franco-American	½
Homestyle, mix, prepared: ¼ cup/Durkee	0
Homestyle, mix, prepared: ¼ cup/French's	½
Homestyle, mix, prepared: ¼ cup/Pillsbury	0
Meatloaf, mix, with roasting bag: 1 pkg/Durkee Roastin' Bag	½
Mushroom:	
Canned: 2 oz./Franco-American	½
Mix, prepared: ¼ cup/French's	½
Onion, mix, prepared: ¼ cup/Durkee	0
Onion, mix, prepared: ¼ cup/French's	½
Onion, mix, prepared: ¼ cup/French's Pan Rich	1½
Onion Pot Roast, mix, with roasting bag: 1 pkg/Durkee Roastin' Bag	½
Pork, mix, prepared: ¼ cup/Durkee	½
Pork, mix, prepared: ¼ cup/French's	½
Pork, pot roast and sparerib mix, with roasting bag: 1 pkg/	
Durkee Roastin' Bag	½
Swiss Steak, mix, prepared: ¼ cup/Durkee	0

	Fat Units
Swiss Steak, mix, with roasting bag: 1 pkg/Durkee Roastin' Bag	½
Turkey Giblet, canned: ½ cup/Howard Johnson's	1
Turkey, mix, prepared: ¼ cup/Durkee	½
Turkey, mix, prepared: ¼ cup/French's	½

HEALTH FOODS

	Fat Units
Granola Bars:	
With cinnamon: 1 bar/Nature Valley	1½
With coconut: 1 bar/Nature Valley	2
With oats and honey: 1 bar/Nature Valley	1½
Peanut: 1 bar/Nature Valley	2
Vegetarian meat substitutes (gluten base unless noted)	
Bologna: ½" slice/Loma Linda	4
Burgers: 1 burger/Loma Linda Sizzle Burgers	3½
Chicken: (4" diameter) ½" slice/Loma Linda	3½
Frankfurters: 1 frank/Loma Linda Big Franks	2
Linketts and Little Links: 1 link/Loma Linda	1
Meatballs: 1 ball/Loma Linda	½
Nuteena: ½" slice/Loma Linda (peanut-butter base)	5
Proteena: ½" slice/Loma Linda (gluten-peanut-butter base)	2
Redi-Burger: ½" slice/Loma Linda	2
Roast Beef: ½" slice/Loma Linda	4
Salami: ½" slice/Loma Linda	4
Sausage: 1 link/Loma Linda Breakfast Links	1
Sausage: 1 piece/Loma Linda Breakfast Sausage	2½
Stew Pac: 2 oz./Loma Linda	½
Swiss Steak: 1 steak/Loma Linda	2½
Tender Bits: 3 bits/Loma Linda	½
Tender Rounds: 1 round/Loma Linda	½
Turkey: ½" slice/Loma Linda	4
Vegeburger: ½ cup/Loma Linda	½
Vegelona: ½" slice/Loma Linda	½
Soy Milk:	
Soyagen, all purpose: 1 cup prepared/Loma Linda	2½
Soyagen, carob: 1 cup prepared/Loma Linda	2½
Soyalac, concentrated: 6 fl. oz. prepared/Loma Linda	2½
Soyalac, powder: 6 fl. oz. prepared/Loma Linda	2½
I-Soyalac, concentrated: 6 fl. oz. prepared/Loma Linda	2½

ICE CREAM AND SHERBET

Ice Cream	
Black Raspberry: ½ cup/Breyers	2
Black Walnut: ½ cup/Meadow Gold	3
Butter Almond: ½ cup/Sealtest	3
Butter Almond, chocolate: ½ cup/Breyers	3
Butter Brickle: ½ cup/Sealtest	2½
Butter Pecan: ½ cup/Meadow Gold	3
Butter Pecan: ½ cup/Sealtest	3½
Caramel Pecan Crunch: ½ cup/Breyers	3
Cherry Nugget: ½ cup/Sealtest	2½

	Fat Units
Cherry Vanilla: ½ cup/Breyers	2½
Cherry Vanilla: ½ cup/Meadow Gold	2
Cherry Vanilla: ½ cup/Sealtest	2
Chocolate: ½ cup/Breyers	3
Chocolate: 4 oz./Howard Johnson's	6½
Chocolate: ½ cup/Meadow Gold	2
Chocolate: ½ cup/Sealtest	2½
Chocolate: ½ cup/Swift's	2
Chocolate Almond: ½ cup/Breyers	3½
Chocolate Almond: ½ cup/Sealtest	3
Chocolate Chip: ½ cup/Meadow Gold	3
Chocolate Chip: ½ cup/Sealtest	3
Chocolate Revel: ½ cup/Meadow Gold	2
Coconut: ½ cup/Sealtest	3
Coffee: ½ cup/Breyers	3
Dutch Chocolate Almond: ½ cup/Breyers	3½
Lemon: ½ cup/Sealtest	2½
Maple Walnut: ½ cup/Sealtest	3
Mint Chocolate Chip: ½ cup/Breyers	3
Peach: ½ cup/Meadow Gold	2
Peach: ½ cup/Sealtest	2
Pineapple: ½ cup/Sealtest	2
Southern Pecan Butterscotch: ½ cup/Breyers	3
Strawberry: ½ cup/Breyers	2
Strawberry: ½ cup/Howard Johnson's	5
Strawberry: ½ cup/Meadow Gold	2
Strawberry: ½ cup/Sealtest	2
Strawberry: ½ cup/Swift's	2
Vanilla: ½ cup/Breyers	3
Vanilla: 4 oz./Howard Johnson's	6½
Vanilla: ½ cup/Meadow Gold	2½
Vanilla: ½ cup/Meadow Gold Golden	2½
Vanilla: ½ cup/Sealtest	2½
Vanilla: ½ cup/Swift's	2½
Vanilla, French: ½ cup/Sealtest	2½
Vanilla Flavored Cherry: ½ cup/Sealtest Royale	2
Vanilla Flavored Red Raspberry: ½ cup/Sealtest Royale	2
Vanilla Fudge Twirl: ½ cup/Breyers	3

Ice Milk

Banana-Strawberry Twirl: ½ cup/Sealtest Light N' Lively	½
Chocolate: ½ cup/Swift's Light n' Easy	1
Chocolate: ½ cup/Sealtest Light N' Lively	½
Coffee: ½ cup/Sealtest Light N' Lively	½
Fudge Twirl: ½ cup/Sealtest Light N' Lively	½
Neapolitan: ½ cup/Sealtest Light N' Lively	½
Peach: ½ cup/Sealtest Light N' Lively	½
Strawberry: ½ cup/Sealtest Light N' Lively	½
Strawberry: ½ cup/Swift's Light 'n Easy	1
Vanilla: ½ cup/Sealtest Light N' Lively	½
Vanilla: ½ cup/Swift's Light 'n Easy	1

Fat Units

Sherbet	
All flavors: ½ cup/various brands	½

ICE CREAM BARS 1 bar or piece

Almond, toasted/Good Humor	5
Banana: 2½ fl. oz. bar/Fudgsicle	1
Chocolate: 2½ fl. oz. bar/Bi-Sicle	1
Chocolate: 2½ fl. oz. bar/Fudgsicle	1
Chocolate Eclair/Good Humor	4½
Creamsicle: 2½ fl. oz. bar	1
Dreamsicle: 2½ fl. oz. bar	1
Icy Whammy, assorted flavors/Good Humor	½
Popsicle, all fruit flavors: 3 fl. oz. bar	½
Sandwich/Good Humor	2
Strawberry Shortcake/Good Humor	4½
Vanilla, chocolate coated/Good Humor	4½
Whammy assorted ice cream/Good Humor	2½
Whammy Chip Crunch/Good Humor	2½

ITALIAN FOODS   See also Pizza and Spaghetti

Cannelloni Florentine, frozen: 13 oz./Weight Watchers	4
Eggplant Parmigiana, frozen: 4 oz./Buitoni	4½
Eggplant Parmigiana, frozen: 13 oz./Weight Watchers	4½
Lasagna:	
Canned: 10 oz./Hormel	5½
Frozen: 4 oz./Buitoni 26 oz. pkg	1½
Frozen, with meat sauce: 4 oz./Buitoni	2
Frozen: 9 oz./Green Giant Boil-in-Bag Entrees	4
Frozen: 10½ oz./Stouffer	5
Frozen: 1 entree/Swanson Hungry-Man	10
Frozen, with cheese, veal, sauce: 13 oz./Weight Watchers	3½
Mix, prepared: ⅕ pkg/Golden Grain Stir-n-Serv	1
Manicotti, frozen, with sauce: 4 oz./Buitoni	2½
Manicotti, frozen, without sauce: 4 oz./Buitoni	3
Ravioli:	
Beef in sauce, canned: 7½ oz./Franco-American	2
Cheese, canned: ½ can/Buitoni	2
Cheese, frozen: 4 oz./Buitoni	4
Meat, canned: ½ can/Buitoni	3
Meat, frozen: 4 oz./Buitoni 40 Count	2½
Meat, frozen: 4 oz./Buitoni Raviolettes	1½
Ravioli Parmigiana, cheese, frozen: 4 oz./Buitoni	11
Ravioli Parmigiana, meat, frozen: 4 oz./Buitoni	3½
Rotini, in tomato sauce, canned: 7½ oz./Franco-American	1½
Rotini & Meatballs, in tomato sauce, canned: 7¼ oz./Franco-American	3
Sausage and peppers, with rigati, frozen: 4 oz./Buitoni	3½
Shells, with sauce, frozen: 4 oz./Buitoni	½
Shrimp Marinara, with shells, frozen: 4 oz./Buitoni	½
Spaghetti with sauce and veal: 1 entree/Swanson "TV"	5½

	Fat Units
Veal Parmigiana:	
Frozen: 7 oz./Green Giant Bake Entrees	6
Frozen, with spaghetti twists: 4 oz./Buitoni	2½
Frozen: 5 oz./Banquet Cookin' Bag	5½
Frozen, with zucchini: 9½ oz./Weight Watchers	3
Ziti, baked, with sauce, frozen: 4 oz./Buitoni	½
Ziti, with veal and sauce, frozen: 13 oz./Weight Watchers	3

MACARONI DISHES

And beef, in tomato sauce, canned: 7½ oz./Franco-American Beefy	3
And beef, with tomato sauce, frozen: 9 oz./Green Giant Boil-in-Bag	3
And beef, with tomatoes, frozen: ½ pkg/Stouffer 11½ oz.	3
And cheese:	
Canned: 7¼ oz./Franco-American	2½
Frozen: 8 oz./Banquet	3½
Frozen: 32 oz./Banquet Supper	16
Frozen: 8 oz./Banquet Cookin' Bag	3½
Frozen: 8 oz./Green Giant Oven Bake Entrees	4½
Frozen: 9 oz./Green Giant Boil-in-Bag Entrees	5½
Frozen: 1 pkg/Morton Casserole	4
Frozen: ½ pkg/Stouffer 12 oz.	4
Frozen: 7 oz./Swanson	3½
Mix, prepared: ¼ pkg/Betty Crocker	5
Mix, prepared: 1 pouch/Betty Crocker Mug-O-Lunch	2
Mix, prepared: ¾ cup/Kraft	4½
And meatballs, in tomato sauce, canned: 7½ oz./Franco-American	
Meatball Mac	3

MAYONNAISE   1 tbsp

Mayonnaise, plain/various brands	4
Flavored/Durkee Famous Sauce	2½
Miracle Whip/Kraft	2½
With relish/Mrs. Filbert's Relish Spread	3
Imitation/Mrs. Filbert's	1½
Imitation/Piedmont	2
Imitation/Weight Watchers	1½

MEAT

Canned, Cured, Processed

Bacon, cooked:	
Hormel Black Label: 1 slice	1
Hormel Red Label: 1 slice	1
Hormel Range Brand: 1 slice	1½
Oscar Mayer: 1 slice	1
Swift Lazy Maple: 1 slice	1
Swift Premium: 1 slice	1
Canadian style: 1 slice/Oscar Mayer	½
Banquet Loaf: 1 slice/Eckrich (8 oz. pkg)	2
Bar-B-Q Loaf: 1 slice/Oscar Mayer	1

	Fat Units
Beef, corned brisket, cooked: 3½ oz./Swift Premium for Oven Roasting	7
Beef, corned, chopped: 1 slice/Eckrich Slender Sliced	½
Beef, chopped: 1 slice/Eckrich Slender Sliced	½
Beef, dried, chunked and formed: ¾ oz./Swift Premium	½
Beef Steaks, breaded, frozen: 4 oz./Hormel	10½
Bologna:	
Eckrich: 1 slice	3
Eckrich thick sliced: 1 slice	5
Hormel/1 oz.	2½
Swift Premium/1 oz.	3
Beef: 1 slice/Eckrich	3
Beef: 1 slice/Oscar Mayer	2½
Coarse ground: 1 oz./Hormel	2
Fine ground: 1 oz./Hormel	2½
Garlic: 1 slice/Eckrich	3
Ring: 2 oz./Eckrich	6½
Ring, garlic: 1 slice/Eckrich	3
Braunschweiger: 1 oz./Oscar Mayer	3
Breakfast Strips: 1 strip/Swift Sizzlean	1½
Frankfurters: 1 frank:	
Eckrich 12 oz. pkg	4
Eckrich Jumbo	6
Eckrich Skinless 16 oz. pkg	4½
Hormel Wieners 12 oz. pkg	3½
Hormel Wieners 16 oz. pkg	4½
Hormel Range Brand Wranglers Smoked Franks	5½
Oscar Mayer Wieners	4½
Beef/Eckrich	4½
Beef/Eckrich Jumbo	6
Beef/Hormel Wieners, 12 oz. pkg	3½
Beef/Hormel Wieners, 16 oz. pkg	4
Beef/Hormel Wranglers Smoked Franks	4
Beef/Oscar Mayer	4½
Frozen, batter-wrapped/Hormel Corn Dogs	4½
Frozen, batter-wrapped/Hormel Tater Dogs	4
Gourmet Loaf: 1 slice/Eckrich	½
Ham, luncheon type:	
Cooked: 1 slice/Eckrich	½
Cooked: 1 oz./Hormel	½
Cooked, smoked: 1 slice/Oscar Mayer	½
Chopped, smoked: 1 slice/Eckrich Slender Sliced	½
Chopped: 1 oz./Hormel	2
Chopped: 2 oz./Hormel 8 lb. can	5½
Chopped: 1 slice/Oscar Mayer	2
Ham Slice, smoked: 4 oz./Oscar Mayer Jubilee	2
Ham Patties: 1 patty/Hormel	6½
Ham Patties: 1 patty/Swift Premium Brown 'n Serve	8½
Ham and Cheese Loaf: 1 slice/Oscar Mayer	2
Honey Loaf: 1 slice/Eckrich	½
Honey Loaf: 1 slice/Oscar Mayer	½
Liver, beef, thin sliced: 2.6 oz./Swift's Tru Tender	2
Liver Cheese: 1 slice/Oscar Mayer	3½

	Fat Units
Luncheon Meat: 1 slice / Oscar Mayer	3
Luncheon Meat, spiced: 1 oz./Hormel	2
Old-Fashioned Loaf: 1 slice/Eckrich	2
Old-Fashioned Loaf: 1 slice/Oscar Mayer	1½
Olive Loaf: 1 slice/Oscar Mayer	1½
Pastrami, chopped: 1 slice/Eckrich Slender Sliced	½
Pepperoni, sliced: 1 oz./Hormel	4½
Pepperoni: 1 oz./Swift	4½
Pickle Loaf: 1 slice/Eckrich, 8 oz. pkg	2½
Pickle and Pimento Loaf: 1 slice/Oscar Mayer	1½
Polish Sausage: 1 link/Eckrich Polska Kielbasa Skinless	5½
Polish Sausage Ring: 2 oz./Eckrich Polska Kielbasa	6½
Polish Sausage Ring: 3 oz./Hormel Kolbase	7½
Polish Sausage, smoked beef: 1 oz./Frito-Lay's	2
Pork Loin, chipped, smoked: 1 slice/Eckrich Slender Sliced	½
Pork Steaks, breaded, frozen: 3 oz./Hormel	5½
Salami:	
Hormel Dairy Hard/1 oz.	3½
Hormel Di Lusso Genoa/1 oz.	4
Oscar Mayer Cotto/1 slice	1½
Oscar Mayer for Beer: 1 slice	1½
Oscar Mayer Hard/1 slice	1
Swift Premium Hard/1 oz.	3
Swift Premium Genoa/1 oz.	3½
Sausage, beef, smoked: 2 oz./Eckrich	6½
Sausage, pork, smoked: 3 oz./Hormel No-Link	9½
Sausage Links:	
Hormel Brown 'n Serve: 1 sausage	2½
Hormel Midget Links: 1 sausage	3½
Hormel Little Sizzlers: 1 sausage	2
Oscar Mayer Little Friers/1 link	2
Swift's The Original/1 link	2½
Swift Premium Brown 'n Serve Kountry Kured/1 link	3
Swift Premium Bacon 'n Sausage/1 link	4
Beef, cooked: 1 link/Swift Premium Brown n' Serve	5½
Sausage Links, smoked:	
Eckrich/1 link, 16 oz. pkg	6
Eckrich Skinless: 1 link	3½
Eckrich Smok-Y-Links/1 link	2½
Hormel Smokies/1 sausage	3
Oscar Mayer/1 link	4
Beef: 1 link/Eckrich Smok-Y-Links	2
Spam: 3 oz./Hormel	8
Spam, with cheese chunks: 3 oz./Hormel	8
Summer Sausage: 1 slice/Oscar Mayer Thuringer Cervelat	2½
Summer Sausage, beef: 1 slice/Oscar Mayer	2
Summer Sausage, beef: 1 oz./Swift Premium	3
Thuringer: 1 oz./Hormel Old Smokehouse	3
Vienna Sausage, canned: 1 piece/Hormel	1½

Fat Units

MEAT ENTREES, CANNED

Beef, with barbecue sauce: 5 oz./Morton House	4
Beef, goulash: 7½ oz. can/Hormel Short Orders	4
Beef, sliced, with gravy: 6¼ oz. can/Morton House	4
Beef stew:	
Canned/Dinty Moore Short Orders: 7½ oz. can	3
Canned/Dinty Moore: 7½ oz. can	3
Canned/Morton House: 8 oz.	4½
Canned/Swanson: 7½ oz.	2½
Hash, beef with potatoes: 7½ oz. can/Dinty Moore Short Orders	4
Hash, corned beef or roast beef, canned: 7½ oz./Mary Kitchen	9
Pork, sliced, with gravy: 6¼ oz./Morton House	4
Salisbury Steak, with mushroom gravy: 4⅙ oz./Morton House	4
Sloppy Joes: 7½ oz. can /Hormel Short Orders	8
Stew, meatball: 6¼ oz./Morton House	6½
Mulligan, stew: 7½ oz. can/Dinty Moore Short Orders	5

MEAT ENTREES, FROZEN

Beef, chipped, creamed: 5 oz./Banquet Cookin' Bag	1½
Beef, chipped, creamed: 5½ oz. pkg/Stouffer	5½
Beef, sliced: 1 entree/Swanson Hungry-Man	3
Beef, sliced, with barbecue sauce: 5 oz./Banquet Cookin' Bag	1
Beef, sliced, with gravy and whipped potatoes: 1 entree/Swanson "TV"	2½
Beef, sliced, with gravy: 5 oz./Banquet Cookin' Bag	1½
Beef, sliced, with gravy: 5 oz./Green Giant Boil-in-Bag Toast Toppers	1½
Beef Stroganoff: 9¾ oz. pkg/Stouffer	7
Green Pepper Steak: 10½ oz. pkg/Stouffer	4½
Meat Loaf:	
Banquet Cookin' Bag: 5 oz.	5½
Morton Country Table: 1 entree	7
With tomato sauce and whipped potatoes: 1 entree/Swanson "TV"	5½
Meatballs, with gravy and whipped potatoes: 1 entree/Swanson "TV"	6
Noodles and Beef: 32 oz./Banquet Buffet Supper	9½
Salisbury Steak:	
Morton Country Table: 1 entree	8½
Stouffer: ½ 12 oz. pkg	5½
With crinkle-cut potatoes: 1 entree/Swanson "TV"	8
With gravy: 5 oz./Banquet Cookin' Bag	6½
With gravy: 7 oz./Green Giant Oven Bake Entrees	6½
With tomato sauce: 9 oz./Green Giant Boil-in-Bag Entrees	9
Sloppy Joes: 5 oz./Banquet Cookin' Bag	4½
Sloppy Joes: 5 oz./Green Giant Boil-in-Bag Toast Toppers	2
Stew, beef: 9 oz./Green Giant Boil-in-Bag Entrees	1
Stew, beef: 10 oz. pkg/Stouffer	6
Stew, beef, with biscuits: 7 oz./Green Giant Oven Bake Entrees	2
Stuffed Cabbage, with beef, in tomato sauce: 7 oz./Green Giant Oven Bake Entrees	4
Stuffed Green Peppers, with beef: 7 oz./Green Giant Oven Bake Entrees	4

	Fat Units
MEAT SPREADS 1 oz. = about ¼ cup	

Chicken, canned: 1 oz./Swanson	2
Chicken: 1 oz./Underwood	1½
Chicken Salad: 1½ oz./Carnation Spreadables	2½
Corned Beef: 1 oz./Underwood	1½
Ham, deviled: 1 oz./Hormel	2
Ham, deviled: 1 oz./Underwood	3
Ham Salad: 1½ oz./Carnation Spreadables	2
Liverwurst: 1 oz./Underwood	3
Roast Beef: 1 oz./Underwood	1½
Sandwich spread:	
Best Foods Spread: 1 tbsp	2
Hellmann's: 1 tbsp	2
Kraft: 1 tbsp	1½
Mrs. Filberts: 1 tbsp	1½
Oscar Mayer: 1 oz.	2
Spam, deviled: 1 oz./Hormel	2½
Tuna or Turkey Salad: 1½ oz./Carnation Spreadables	2

MEAT SUBSTITUTES

Breakfast Links: 1 link/Morningstar Farms	1½
Breakfast Patties: 1 pattie/Morningstar Farms	2½
Breakfast Strips: 1 strip/Morningstar Farms	1½
Grillers: one griller/Morningstar Farms	5
Luncheon slices: 1 slice/Morningstar Farms	½

MEXICAN FOODS

Beans, refried, canned, ½ cup/Ortega	1½
Burritos, beef, canned: 4 oz./Hormel	3
Chili Con Carne, canned:	
With beans, low sodium: 7¾ oz./Campbell	5½
With beans: 7½ oz./Hormel	6½
With beans: 7½ oz./Morton House	6½
With beans: 7¾ oz./Swanson	5½
Without beans: 7½ oz./Hormel	9
Without beans: 7½ oz./Morton House	7
Chili Mac, canned: 7½ oz./Hormel Short Orders	3½
Enchiladas:	
Frozen, beef, with sauce: 6 oz./Banquet Cookin' Bag	2½
Frozen, beef, with gravy: 3 enchiladas/El Chico	11½
Queso Dinner, frozen: 1 dinner/El Chico	7
Saltillo Dinner, frozen: 1 dinner/El Chico	10½
Taco Shell: 1 shell/Ortega	½
Tacos, beef, frozen: 3 tacos/El Chico	6
Tamales, beef, canned: 1 tamale/Hormel	2
Tamales, beef, in jar: 2 tamales/Swift Derby	3

Fat Units

MUFFINS: ENGLISH AND SWEET   1 muffin unless noted

Apple Cinnamon, refrigerator, to bake/Pillsbury	2
Apple Cinnamon, mix, prepared/Betty Crocker	2
Banana Nut, mix, prepared: Betty Crocker Chiquita	2½
Blueberry:	
Thomas' Toast-R-Cakes	1½
Frozen/Morton	1
Frozen/Pepperidge Farm	1½
Mix, prepared/Betty Crocker	1½
Bran/Oroweat Bran'nola	½
Bran/Thomas' Toast-R-Cakes	1
Corn	
Thomas'	3
Thomas' Toast-R-Cakes	1½
Frozen/Morton	1½
Frozen/Pepperidge Farm	2
Frozen/Thomas' Toast-R-Cakes	1½
Mix, prepared/Betty Crocker	2
Mix, prepared/Flako	1½
Refrigerator to bake/Pillsbury	2
English/various brands	½
Pineapple, mix, prepared/Betty Crocker	1
Raisin/Oroweat	½
Raisin/Wonder Rounds	1
Raisin Bran, frozen/Pepperidge Farm	2
Wild Blueberry, mix, prepared/Duncan Hines	1

NOODLE DISHES

Almondine, mix, prepared: ¼ pkg/Betty Crocker	4
With Beef-Flavored Sauce, mix, prepared: 1 pouch/Betty Crocker Mug-O-Lunch	1
With Beef Sauce, mix, prepared: ½ cup/Pennsylvania Dutch Brand	1
With Butter Sauce, mix, prepared: ½ cup/Pennsylvania Dutch Brand	1½
With Cheese, mix, prepared: ⅕ pkg/Noodle-Roni Parmesano	1
With Cheese Sauce, mix, prepared: ½ cup/Pennsylvania Dutch Brand	1
With Chicken Sauce, mix, prepared: ½ cup/Pennsylvania Dutch Brand	1
Romanoff, frozen: ⅓ pkg/Stouffer	3
Romanoff, mix, prepared: ¼ pkg/Betty Crocker	4
Stroganoff, mix: 2 oz./Pennsylvania Dutch Brand	1
Stroganoff, mix, prepared: ¼ pkg/Betty Crocker	4
With Tuna, frozen: ½ pkg/Stouffer 11½ oz.	3

PANCAKES, WAFFLES, AND SIMILAR BREAKFAST FOODS

Breakfast, frozen, French toast, with sausages: 1 entree/Swanson "TV"	6
Breakfast, frozen, pancakes and sausages: 1 entree/Swanson "TV"	9
Breakfast, frozen, scrambled eggs, with sausage and coffee cake: 1 entree/Swanson "TV"	11
Breakfast Bars: 1 bar/Carnation	3½

	Fat Units
Breakfast Squares: 1 bar/General Mills	3
Crepes, mix, prepared: 2 crepes 6″ diameter/Aunt Jemima	1½
French Toast, frozen: 1 slice/Downyflake	2½
French Toast, frozen: 1 slice/Aunt Jemima	1
French Toast, with cinnamon, frozen: 1 slice/Aunt Jemima Cinnamon Swirl	1
Fritters, apple or corn, frozen: 1 fritter/Mrs. Paul's	2
Pancakes, frozen: 1 pancake/Downyflake	1
Pancake Batter, frozen: 3 cakes 4″ diameter/Aunt Jemima	2
Pancake Batter, frozen: 3 cakes 4″ diameter/Aunt Jemima Blueberry	2
Pancake Batter, frozen: 3 cakes 4″ diameter/Aunt Jemima Buttermilk	2
Pancake, mix, prepared:	
Hungry Jack Complete: 3 cakes, 4″ diameter	2
Hungry Jack Extra Lights: 3 cakes 4″ diameter	2
Tillie Lewis/3 cakes 4″ diameter	1
Blueberry: 3 cakes 4″ diameter/Hungry Jack	5½
Buttermilk: 3 cakes 4″ diameter/Betty Crocker	3
Buttermilk: 3 cakes 4″ diameter/Betty Crocker Complete	2
Buttermilk: 3 cakes 4″ diameter/Hungry Jack Complete	2
Butermilk: 3 cakes 4″ diameter/Hungry Jack	4
Pancake-waffle mix prepared:	
Aunt Jemima Original: 3 cakes 4″ diameter	3
Aunt Jemima Complete: 3 cakes 4″ diameter	2
Log Cabin complete: 3 cakes 4″ diameter	2
Log Cabin Regular: 3 cakes 4″ diameter	2
Buckwheat: 3 cakes 4″ diameter/Aunt Jemima	3
Buttermilk: 3 cakes 4″ diameter/Aunt Jemima	4
Buttermilk: 3 cakes 4″ diameter/Aunt Jemima Complete	2½
Whole wheat: 3 cakes 4″ diameter/Aunt Jemima	3
Waffles, frozen:	
Aunt Jemima Jumbo Original: 1 waffle	1
Downyflake, regular and jumbo: 1 waffle	1
Downyflake Hot 'n Buttery: 1 waffle	1
Eggo: 1 waffle	2

PASTRY

Donuts, frozen: 1 donut	
Morton Mini	2
Bavarian or Boston Creme/Morton	3
Chocolate Iced or Glazed/Morton	2½
Jelly/Morton	3
Dumplings, apple, frozen: 1 dumpling/Pepperidge Farm	6
Pie-Tarts, frozen: 1 tart	
Apple, Blueberry, Cherry/Pepperidge Farm	5½
Lemon or Raspberry/Pepperidge Farm	6½
Strudel, apple, frozen: 3 oz./Pepperidge Farm	4½
Turnovers: 1 turnover	
Frozen/Pepperidge Farm	7
Refrigerator/Pillsbury	3

Fat Units

PIES

Frozen: 1 whole pie

Apple:

Banquet: 20 oz.	20½
Morton: 24 oz.	27½
Mrs. Smith's: 8″	32
Mrs. Smith's (natural juice): 8″	48½
Dutch/Mrs. Smith's: 8″	27½
Tart/Mrs. Smith's: 8″	19
Banana Cream/Mrs. Smith's Light: 13.8 oz.	25½
Banana Cream/Banquet: 14 oz.	20½
Banana Cream/Morton: 16 oz.	21
Banana Cream/Morton Mini: 3.5 oz.	5
Banana Cream/Mrs. Smith's: 8″	23½

Blueberry:

Banquet: 20 oz.	21½
Morton: 24 oz.	29½
Morton Mini: 8 oz.	9
Mrs. Smith's: 8″	29½
Mrs. Smith's (with natural juice): 8″	36
Boston Cream/Mrs. Smith's: 8″	27½

Cherry:

Banquet: 20 oz.	19
Morton: 24 oz.	29½
Morton Mini: 8 oz.	9
Mrs. Smith's: 8″	29½
Mrs. Smith's (natural juice): 8″	34
Chocolate/Mrs. Smith's Light: 13.8 oz.	25½
Chocolate Cream/Banquet: 14 oz.	19½
Chocolate Cream/Morton: 16 oz.	25½
Chocolate Cream/Morton Mini: 3.5 oz.	5½
Chocolate Cream/Mrs. Smith's: 8″	25½
Coconut/Mrs. Smith's Light: 13.8 oz.	25½
Coconut Cream/Banquet: 14 oz.	21½
Coconut Cream/Morton: 16 oz.	23½
Coconut Cream/Morton Mini: 3.5 oz.	5½
Coconut Cream/Mrs. Smith's: 8″	23½
Coconut Custard/Banquet: 20 oz.	16½
Coconut Custard/Morton Mini: 6.5 oz.	5½
Coconut Custard/Mrs. Smith's: 8″	25½
Custard/Banquet: 20 oz.	14
Egg Custard/Mrs. Smith's: 8″	21
Lemon/Mrs. Smith's: 8″	36
Lemon Cream/Banquet: 14 oz.	18
Lemon Cream/Morton: 16 oz.	21
Lemon Cream/Morton Mini: 3.5 oz.	5
Lemon Cream/Mrs. Smith's: 8″	23½
Lemon Krunch/Mrs. Smith's: 8″	34
Lemon Meringue/Mrs. Smith's: 8″	21
Lemon Yogurt/Mrs. Smith's: 15.6 oz.	19

	Fat Units
Mincemeat/Banquet: 20 oz.	20
Mince/Morton: 24 oz.	29½
Mince/Morton Mini: 8 oz.	9
Mince/Mrs. Smith's: 8"	29½
Neapolitan Cream/Morton: 16 oz.	23½
Neapolitan Cream/Mrs. Smith's: 8"	25½
Peach/Banquet: 20 oz.	21
Peach/Morton: 24 oz.	27½
Peach/Morton Mini: 8 oz.	9
Peach/Mrs. Smith's: 8"	29½
Peach (natural juice)/Mrs. Smith's: 8"	34
Pecan/Morton Mini: 6.5 oz.	10
Pecan/Mrs. Smith's: 8"	42½
Pineapple Cheese/Mrs. Smith's: 8"	23½
Pumpkin/Banquet: 20 oz.	14½
Pumpkin/Morton: 24 oz.	17
Pumpkin/Morton Mini: 8 oz.	5
Pumpkin/Mrs. Smith's: 8"	21
Raisin/Mrs. Smith's: 8"	29½
Strawberry Cream/Banquet: 14 oz.	17½
Strawberry Cream/Morton: 16 oz.	21
Strawberry Cream/Mrs. Smith's: 8"	23½
Strawberry-Rhubarb/Mrs. Smith's: 8"	29½
Strawberry-Rhubarb (natural juice)/Mrs. Smith's: 8"	34
Strawberry-Rhubarb (natural juice)/Mrs. Smith's: 9"	48½
Strawberry Yogurt/Mrs. Smith's: 15.6 oz.	21

PIE CRUSTS AND PASTRY SHELLS

Pastry Sheets, frozen: 1 sheet/Pepperidge Farm	16
Patty Shells, frozen: 1 shell/Pepperidge Farm	6½
Pie Crust, mix, prepared: double crust/Betty Crocker	45
Pie Crust, mix, prepared: 1 whole crust/Flako	29½
Pie Crust, mix, prepared: double crust/Pillsbury	38
Pie Crust, stick: 1 stick/Betty Crocker	25½
Pie Shells, deep, frozen: 1 shell/Pepperidge Farm	12½
Pie Shell, shallow bottom, frozen: 1 bottom/Pepperidge Farm	11½
Pie Shells, top, frozen: 1 top/Pepperidge Farm	20
Tart Shells, frozen: 1 shell/Pepperidge Farm	2

PIE FILLING

Apple: 21 oz. can/Wilderness	6
Apple, French: 21 oz. can/Wilderness	6
Apricot: 21 oz. can/Wilderness	7
Blueberry: 21 oz. can/Wilderness	6
Cherry: 21 oz. can/Wilderness	6
Key Lime, mix, prepared: ½ cup/Royal Cooked	1½
Lemon: 22 oz. can/Wilderness	8½
Lemon, mix, prepared: ½ cup/Royal Cooked	1½
Mincemeat: ⅓ cup/None Such	1½
Mince: 22 oz. can/Wilderness	10½

	Fat Units
Peach: 21 oz. can/Wilderness	6
Pumpkin, canned: 1 cup/Stokely-Van Camp	3½
Raisin: 22 oz. can/Wilderness	7
Strawberry: 21 oz. can/Wilderness	7

PIZZA 1 whole pizza unless noted

Beef and Cheese, frozen: El Chico Mexican	21
Canadian Bacon, frozen: Totino's Party	7
Cheese:	
Frozen: 4 oz./Buitoni	3
Frozen: 7 oz./Celeste	6½
Frozen: Celeste Sicilian Style 20 oz. size	15½
Frozen: Jeno's 13 oz. size	9
Frozen: La Pizzeria 20 oz.	15½
Frozen: ½ pkg/Stouffer	4½
Frozen: Totino's	12½
Mix, prepared: Jeno's	8
Chili and Cheese, frozen: El Chico Mexican	20½
Combination:	
Frozen: Celeste Deluxe 9 oz. size	11½
Frozen: Jeno's Deluxe 23 oz. size	27½
Frozen: La Pizzeria 13.5 oz.	15½
Frozen: ½ pkg/Stouffer Deluxe	6½
Frozen, deep crust: Totino's Classic	14
Frozen: Totino's Classic	34
Hamburger, frozen: Jeno's	10
Hamburger, frozen: Totino's	15½
Open Face, frozen: 4 oz./Buitoni	2
Pepperoni:	
Frozen: Celeste 7½ oz. size	9
Frozen: Jeno's 13 oz. size	10½
Frozen: La Pizzeria 21 oz.	22½
Frozen: ½ pkg/Stouffer	6½
Frozen, deep crust: Totino's	12½
Mix, prepared: Jeno's	14
Refried Bean and Cheese, frozen: El Chico Mexican	16
Regular, mix, prepared: Jeno's	8½
Sausage:	
Frozen: Celeste 8 oz. size	10½
Frozen: Jeno's 13 oz. size	11½
Frozen: La Pizzeria 13 oz.	16
Frozen, deep crust: Totino's Classic	12½
Frozen: Totino's Crisp Party	16
Mix, prepared: Jeno's	15½
And Mushroom, frozen: Celeste 9 oz. size	10

POT PIES

Frozen: 1 whole pie
Beef:

Banquet: 8 oz.	7
Morton: 8 oz.	5½

	Fat Units
Stouffer: 10 oz.	13½
Swanson: 8 oz.	8
Chicken:	
Banquet: 8 oz.	8
Morton: 8 oz.	7
Stouffer: 10 oz.	10
Swanson: 8 oz.	9
Tuna/Banquet: 8 oz.	8
Tuna/Morton: 8 oz.	6½
Turkey:	
Banquet: 8 oz.	7½
Morton: 8 oz.	7½
Stouffer: 10 oz.	9
Swanson: 8 oz.	9

POULTRY DISHES

Chicken à la King, canned: 5¼ oz./Swanson	4
Chicken à la King, frozen: 5 oz./Banquet Cookin' Bag	1½
Chicken à la King, frozen: 5 oz./Green Giant Toast Toppers	3½
Chicken à la King, frozen: 1 pkg/Stouffer 9½ oz.	4
Chicken, boned white chunk, canned: 2½ oz./Swanson	2
Chicken, boned, with broth, canned: 2½ oz./Swanson	2
Chicken, chopped, pressed: 1 slice/Eckrich Slender Sliced	1
Chicken and Biscuits, frozen: 7 oz./Green Giant Oven Bake	5½
Chicken Breast Parmigiana, frozen: 9 oz./Weight Watchers	3
Chicken, creamed, frozen: 1 pkg/Stouffer 6½ oz.	8
Chicken Creole, frozen: Weight Watchers 13 oz.	1½
Croquette, chicken, with sauce, frozen: 12 oz./Howard Johnson's	12
Chicken Divan, frozen: 1 pkg/Stouffer 8½ oz.	8
Chicken with Dumplings, canned: 7½ oz./Swanson	4
Chicken, escalloped, frozen: ½ pkg/Stouffer 11½ oz.	5½
Chicken, fried:	
Frozen: 6.4 oz./Morton	6½
Frozen, assorted pieces: 3.2 edible oz./Swanson	6
With Whipped Potatoes: 1 entree/Swanson "TV" 7 oz.	8
Chicken Livers with Chopped Broccoli, frozen: 10½ oz./Weight Watchers	2
Chicken Nibbles, with french fries: 1 entree/Swanson "TV"	7
Chicken and Noodles, frozen: 32 oz./Banquet Buffet Supper	7½
Chicken and Noodles, frozen: 9 oz./Green Giant Boil-In-Bag	3½
Chicken Stew, canned: 7½ oz./Swanson	2½
Chicken, white meat, with peas, onion, frozen: 9 oz./Weight Watchers	4
Turkey, boned, with broth, canned: 2½ oz./Swanson	2
Turkey Slices:	
Canned, with gravy: 6¼ oz./Morton House	2
Frozen entree: 8¾ oz./Swanson "TV"	3
Frozen, with giblet gravy: 5 oz./Banquet Cookin' Bag	1½
Frozen with gravy: 5 oz./Green Giant Toast Toppers	1½
Turkey Tetrazzini, frozen: ½ pkg/Stouffer 12 oz.	5
Turkey Tetrazzini, with mushrooms, red peppers, frozen: 13 oz./ Weight Watchers	3
Turkey, smoked, chopped: 1 slice/Eckrich Slender Sliced	1

Fat Units

PUDDINGS

All flavors, canned: ½ cup/Betty Crocker	2½
All flavors, canned: 5 oz./Del Monte	2½
All flavors, mix prepared with whole milk: ½ cup/various brands	2½
Plum, canned, ready to serve: ½ cup/R & R	3

RICE DISHES

Beef-Flavored, mix, prepared: ⅙ pkg/Rice-A-Roni	½
Beef-Flavored, mix, prepared: ½ cup/Minute Rice Rib Roast	1½
Beef-Flavored, mix, prepared: ½ cup/Uncle Ben's	½
With Bell Peppers and Parsley, frozen: 1 cup/Green Giant Verdi	2½
With Broccoli, in cheese sauce, frozen: 1 cup/Green Giant	3
Chicken-Flavored, mix, prepared: ⅕ pkg/Rice-A-Roni	½
Chicken-Flavored, mix, prepared: ½ cup/Uncle Ben's	½
Curried, mix, prepared: 1 cup/Uncle Ben's	½
Fried, mix, prepared: ½ cup/Minute	2
With Green Beans and Almonds, frozen: 1 cup/Green Giant Continental	3
And Peas, with mushrooms, frozen: 2.3 oz./Birds Eye Combinations	0
With Peas and Mushrooms, frozen: 1 cup/Green Giant Medley	2
Pilaf, mix, prepared: 1 cup/Uncle Ben's	½
Pilaf, with mushrooms and onions, frozen: 1 cup/Green Giant	1½
Poultry-Flavored, mix, prepared: ½ cup/Minute Drumstick	2
Spanish, mix, prepared: ½ cup/Minute	1½
Spanish, mix, prepared: ⅙ pkg/Rice-A-Roni	½
Spanish, mix, prepared: 1 cup/Uncle Ben's	½
White and Wild, with bean sprouts, frozen: 1 cup/Green Giant Oriental	2
White and Wild, with peas, frozen: 1 cup/Green Giant Medley	4

ROLLS, SWEET   1 roll unless noted

Caramel, refrigerated/Pillsbury Danish	3
Cinnamon, refrigerated/Ballard	1
Cinnamon with Icing, refrigerated/Hungry Jack Butter Tastin'	2½
Cinnamon with Icing, refrigerated/Pillsbury	1½
Cinnamon-Raisin, refrigerated/Pillsbury Danish	2½
Honey Buns, frozen/Morton	4
Honey Buns, frozen/Morton Mini	2
Orange, refrigerated/Pillsbury Danish	1½

SALAD DRESSINGS   Bottled unless noted

Mrs. Filbert's Salad Dressing: 1 tbsp	2
Nu Made Salad Dressing: 1 tbsp	2½
Piedmont Salad Dressing: 1 tbsp	1½
Sultana Salad Dressing: 1 tbsp	2
Avocado: 1 tbsp/Kraft	2½
Blue Cheese:	
Kraft Chunkey: 1 tbsp	
Kraft Low Calorie: 1 tbsp	
Kraft Roka: 1 tbsp	

	Fat Units
Seven Seas Real: 1 tbsp	2½
Wish-Bone Chunky: 1 tbsp	3
Mix, prepared: 1 tbsp/Weight Watchers	½
Caesar:	
Kraft Golden: 1 tbsp	2½
Pfeiffer: 1 tbsp	3
Seven Seas: 1 tbsp	2½
Wish-Bone: 1 tbsp	3
Chef Style: 1 tbsp/Kraft Low Calorie	½
Coleslaw Dressing: 1 tbsp/Kraft	2
Coleslaw Dressing: 1 tbsp/Kraft Low Calorie	½
Cucumber, creamy: 1 tbsp/Kraft	3
Cucumber, creamy: 1 tbsp/Kraft Low Calorie	1
French:	
Kraft: 1 tbsp	2
Kraft Casino Garlic: 1 tbsp	2
Kraft Catalina: 1 tbsp	2
Kraft Herb and Garlic: 1 tbsp	3½
Kraft Low Calorie: 1 tbsp	½
Kraft Miracle: 1 tbsp	2
Nu Made Low Calorie: 1 tbsp	½
Nu Made Savory: 1 tbsp	2
Nu Made Zesty: 1 tbsp	2½
Pfeiffer: 1 tbsp	2
Pfeiffer Low-Cal: 1 tbsp	½
Seven Seas Family Style: 1 tbsp	2
Seven Seas Low Calorie: 1 tbsp	½
Wish-Bone: 1 tbsp	2
Wish-Bone Low Calorie: 1 tbsp	½
Seven Seas Creamy: 1 tbsp	2
Mix, prepared: 1 tbsp/Weight Watchers	0
French Style: 1 tbsp/Kraft Low Calorie	½
Garlic, creamy: 1 tbsp/Kraft	2
Garlic, creamy: 1 tbsp/Wish-Bone	3
Green Goddess:	
Kraft: 1 tbsp	3
Nu Made: 1 tbsp	2
Herbs and Spices: 1 tbsp/Seven Seas	2
Italian:	
Kraft: 1 tbsp	3
Kraft Golden Blend: 1 tbsp	2½
Kraft Low Calorie: 1 tbsp	0
Seven Seas: 1 tbsp	3
Seven Seas Viva: 1 tbsp	3
Wish-Bone: 1 tbsp	3
Wish-Bone Low Calorie: 1 tbsp	½
Creamy: 1 tbsp/Kraft	2
Creamy: 1 tbsp/Seven Seas	2½
Creamy: 1 tbsp/Weight Watchers	2
Mix, prepared: 1 tbsp/Good Seasons Low Calorie	0
Mix, prepared: 1 tbsp/Weight Watchers	0
Creamy, mix, prepared: 1 tbsp/Weight Watchers	0

	Fat Units
May Lo Naise: 1 tbsp/Tillie Lewis	1
Oil and Vinegar: 1 tbsp/Kraft	2
Onion: 1 tbsp/Wish-Bone California	3
Russian:	
Kraft Low Calorie: 1 tbsp	½
Nu Made: 1 tbsp	2
Pfeiffer: 1 tbsp	2½
Pfeiffer Low-Cal: 1 tbsp	½
Seven Seas Creamy: 1 tbsp	3
Weight Watchers: 1 tbsp	2
Wish-Bone: 1 tbsp	1
Wish-Bone Low Calorie: 1 tbsp	½
Creamy: 1 tbsp/Kraft	2
Mix, prepared: 1 tbsp/Weight Watchers	0
Salad Secret: 1 tbsp/Kraft	2
Sour Treat: 1 oz./Friendship	1½
Spin Blend: 1 tbsp/Hellman's	2
Thousand Island:	
Kraft: 1 tbsp	2
Kraft Low Calorie: 1 tbsp	½
Pfeiffer: 1 tbsp	2½
Pfeiffer: 1 tbsp	½
Seven Seas: 1 tbsp	2
Weight Watchers: 1 tbsp	2
Wish-Bone: 1 tbsp	2½
Wish-Bone Low Calorie: 1 tbsp	½
Mix, prepared: 1 tbsp/Weight Watchers	½
Yogonaise: 1 tbsp/Henri's	2
Yogowhip: 1 tbsp/Henri's	2
Yogurt: 1 tbsp/Henri's	½

SAUCES

	Fat Units
A la King, mix, prepared: ½ cup/Durkee	1½
Barbecue, bottled or canned:	
French's: 1 tbsp	0
Cheese, mix, prepared: ½ cup/Durkee	3½
Cheese, mix, prepared: ¼ cup/French's	1½
Hollandaise, mix, prepared: ¾ cup/Durkee	5
Hollandaise, mix, prepared: 3 tbsp/French's	1½
Horseradish Sauce: 1 tbsp/Kraft	2
Italian, canned: 2 fl. oz. /Contadina Cookbook	½
Italian, red, in jar: 5 oz./Ragú	½
Lemon-Butter Flavored, mix, prepared: 1 tbsp/Weight Watchers	0
Mushroom Steak, canned: 1 oz./Dawn Fresh	0
Pizza, canned: 4 oz./Buitoni	2
Pizza, in jar: 5 oz./Ragú	2
Sour Cream, mix, prepared: ⅔ cup/Durkee	2½
Sour cream, mix, prepared: 2½ tbsp/French's	2
Spaghetti:	
Canned: 4 oz./Buitoni	1½
In Jar: 5 oz./Ragú plain and Extra Thick	2

	Fat Units
Mix, prepared: ½ cup/Durkee	½
Mix, prepared: ⅝ cup/French's Italian style	1½
Mix, prepared: 4 fl. oz./Spatini	3
Clam, canned: 5 oz./Ragú	2
Clam, red, canned: 4 oz./Buitoni	1½
Clam, white, canned: 4 oz./Buitoni	4
Marinara, canned: 4 oz./Buitoni	2
Marinara, in jar: 5 oz./Ragú	2
Meat-Flavor, canned: 4 oz./Buitoni	3
Meat-Flavor, in jar: 5 oz./Ragú	2½
Meat-Flavor, in jar: 5 oz./Ragú extra thick	2½
With Mushrooms, canned: 4 oz./Buitoni	2
With Mushrooms, in jar: 5 oz./Ragú plain and extra thick	2
With Mushrooms, mix, prepared: ⅔ cup/Durkee	½
With Mushrooms, mix, prepared: ⅝ cup/French's	1½
Pepperoni flavor, in jar: 5 oz./Ragú	2½
Stroganoff: mix, prepared: ⅓ cup/French's	2
Sweet and Sour, canned: 2 fl. oz./Contadina Cookbook	1
Sweet and Sour, canned: 1 cup/La Choy	6
Sweet and Sour, mix, prepared: 1 cup/Durkee	3
Sweet and Sour, mix, prepared: ½ cup/French's	½
Swiss Steak, canned: 2 fl. oz./Contadina Cookbook	0
Teriyaki, mix, prepared: 2 tbsp/French's	0
Tomato, canned:	
Contadina: 1 cup	½
Del Monte: 1 cup	½
Hunt's: 4 oz.	½
Hunt's Prima Salsa Regular: 4 oz.	1
Hunt's Special: 4 oz.	½
Stokely-Van Camp: 1 cup	½
With Bits: 4 oz./Hunt's	½
With Cheese: 4 oz./Hunt's	½
With Herbs: 4 oz./Hunt's	1½
Meat-Flavor: 4 oz./Hunt's Prima Salsa	1
With Mushrooms: 1 cup/Del Monte	½
With Mushrooms: 4 oz./Hunt's	½
Mushroom: 4 oz./Hunt's Prima Salsa	1
With Onions: 1 cup/Del Monte	½
With Onions: 4 oz./Hunt's	½
With Tidbits: 1 cup/Del Monte	½
White, mix, prepared: ½ cup/Durkee	2½

SEAFOOD, CANNED AND FROZEN

	Fat Units
Clams:	
Chopped or minced, canned: 1 cup	½
Fried, frozen: 2½ oz./Mrs. Paul's	5½
Cakes, frozen: 1 cake/Mrs. Paul's Thins	2½
Deviled, frozen: 1 cake/Mrs. Paul's	3½
Sticks, frozen: 1 stick/Mrs. Paul's	½
Crab Cakes, frozen: 1 cake/Mrs. Paul's Thins	2½
Crabs, deviled, frozen: 1 cake/Mrs. Paul's	2½

	Fat Units
Fish, frozen:	
Cakes: 1 cake /Mrs. Paul's	1½
Cakes: 1 cake/Mrs. Paul's Thins	3
Fillets, buttered: 1 fillet (2½ oz.)/Mrs. Paul's	4½
Fillets, fried: 1 fillet (2 oz.)/Mrs. Paul's	1½
Fillets, in light batter: 1 fillet/Mrs. Paul's	2½
Sticks: 1 stick/Mrs. Paul's	½
Sticks, in light batter, fried: 1 stick/Mrs. Paul's	1
Flounder, with lemon butter, frozen: 4½ oz./Mrs. Paul's	3
Haddock, fried, frozen: 1 fillet 2 oz./Mrs. Paul's	1½
Perch, fried, frozen: 1 fillet 2 oz./Mrs. Paul's	2½
Salmon, canned: ½ cup/various brands	3
Sardines, sauce or oil: 1 oz./various brands	1½
Scallops, fried, frozen: 3½ oz./Mrs. Paul's	3
Seafood croquettes, frozen: 1 cake/Mrs. Paul's	2
Shrimp:	
Fried, frozen: 3 oz./Mrs. Paul's	4
Cakes, frozen: 1 cake/Mrs. Paul's	2
Sticks, frozen: 1 stick/Mrs. Paul's	½
Sole, with lemon butter, frozen: 4½ oz./Mrs. Paul's	3
Tuna, canned:	
In Oil: ½ cup/various brands	2½
In Water: ½ cup/various brands	1

SEAFOOD ENTREES—FROZEN

Crepes, clam: 5½ oz./Mrs. Paul's	6
Crepes, crab or shrimp: 5½ oz./Mrs. Paul's	4
Crepes, scallop: 5½ oz./Mrs. Paul's	3
Croquette, shrimp, with Newburg sauce: 12 oz./Howard Johnson's	13½
Fish au Gratin: 5 oz./Mrs. Paul's	4
Fish 'n' Chips: 1 entree/Swanson "TV"	5
Fish 'n' Chips, in light batter, fried: 7 oz./Mrs. Paul's	5½
Fish Parmesan: 5 oz./Mrs. Paul's	4
Flounder, with chopped broccoli, cauliflower and red peppers:	
8½ oz./Weight Watchers	½
Haddock, with stuffing and spinach: 8¾ oz./Weight Watchers	½
Perch, ocean, with chopped broccoli: 8½ oz./Weight Watchers	2
Scallops, with butter and cheese: 7 oz./Mrs. Paul's	4
Sole, with peas, mushrooms and lobster sauce: 9½ oz./Weight Watchers	1
Shrimp and Scallops Mariner: 10¼ oz. pkg/Stouffer	5½
Tuna, creamed, with peas: 5 oz./Green Giant Toast Toppers	3
Turbot, with peas and carrots: 8 oz./Weight Watchers	5½

SOUPS

Alphabet Vegetable, mix, prepared: 6 fl. oz./Lipton Cup-A-Soup	½
Asparagus, cream of, condensed, prepared: 10 oz./Campbell	2
Bean, canned:	
Semi-Condensed, prepared: 1 can/Campbell Soup for One	3
With Bacon, condensed, prepared: 10 oz./Campbell	2
Black, condensed, prepared: 10 oz./Campbell	½

	Fat Units
Black, ready to serve: ½ can/Crosse & Blackwell	½
With Ham, ready to serve: 1 can (10¾ oz.)/Campbell Chunky	4
With Ham, ready to serve: ½ can (9½ oz.)/Campbell	3½
With Hot Dogs, condensed, prepared: 10 oz./Campbell	3
Beef:	
Condensed, prepared: 10 oz./Campbell	1
Ready to serve: ½ can (9½ oz.)/Campbell Chunky	2½
Ready to serve, individual service size: 1 can (10¾ oz.)/	
Campbell Chunky	3
Flavor, mix, prepared: 8 oz./Lipton Lite-Lunch	2½
Cabbage, condensed, prepared: 8 oz./Manischewitz	1
Mushroom, mix, prepared: 8 fl. oz./Lipton	½
Noodle, condensed, prepared: 10 oz./Campbell	1
Noodle, mix, prepared: 1 envelope/Souptime	½
Borscht, condensed, prepared: 8 oz./Manischewitz	0
Bouillon Cubes: 1 cube/various brands	0
Broth:	
Beef, condensed, prepared: 10 oz./Campbell	½
Beef, canned: 6¾ oz./Swanson	½
Beef: 1 packet/Herb-Ox	0
Beef, mix: 1 packet/Weight Watchers Broth and Seasoning Mix	0
Chicken, condensed, prepared: 10 oz./Campbell	1
Chicken, canned: 6¾ oz./Swanson	½
Chicken: 1 packet/Herb-Ox	0
Chicken, mix, prepared: 6 fl. oz./Lipton Cup-A-Broth	½
Chicken, mix: 1 packet/Weight Watchers	0
Celery, cream of, condensed, prepared: 10 oz./Campbell	2½
Cheddar Cheese, condensed, prepared: 10 oz./Campbell	4
Chickarina, canned, ready to serve: 8 fl. oz./Progresso	2
Chicken:	
Canned, ready to serve: ½ can (9½ oz.)/Campbell Chunky	2½
Flavor, mix, prepared: 8 oz./Lipton Lite-Lunch	3
Alphabet, condensed, prepared: 10 oz./Campbell	1
Barley, condensed, prepared: 8 oz./Manischewitz	1½
Cream of, condensed, prepared: 10 oz./Campbell	3
Cream of, mix, prepared: 6 fl. oz./Lipton Cup-A-Soup	1
Cream of, mix, prepared: 1 envelope/Souptime	2
With Dumplings, condensed, prepared: 10 oz./Campbell	2½
Gumbo, condensed, prepared: 10 oz./Campbell	½
Noodle, condensed, prepared: 10 oz./Campbell	1
Noodle, condensed, prepared: 8 oz./Manischewitz	1
Noodle, mix, prepared: 6 fl. oz./Lipton	½
Rice, condensed, prepared: 10 oz./Campbell	1
Rice, mix, prepared: 8 fl. oz./Lipton	½
With Stars, condensed, prepared: 10 oz./Campbell	1
Vegetable, condensed, prepared: 10 oz./Campbell	1½
Vegetable, canned, ready to serve: ½ can (9½ oz.)/Campbell Chunky	2
Vegetable, condensed, prepared: 8 oz./Manischewitz	1
Vegetable, mix, prepared: 6 fl. oz./Lipton Cup-A-Soup	½
Chili Beef, condensed, prepared: 10 oz./Campbell	3
Chili Beef, ready to serve: ½ can (9¾ oz.)/Campbell Chunky	2

	Fat Units
Chowder:	
Clam, prepared: 1 cup/Howard Johnson's	3
Clam, ready to serve: 8 fl. oz./Progresso	½
Clam, Manhattan, condensed, prepared: 10 oz./Campbell	1
Clam, Manhattan, ready to serve: ½ can/Crosse & Blackwell	½
Clam, Manhattan, condensed, prepared: 7 oz./Snow's	2
Clam, New England, ready to serve: ½ can/Crosse & Blackwell	1
Clam, New England, condensed, prepared: 7 oz./Snow's	2
Consomme (Beef), condensed, prepared: 10 oz./Campbell	½
Consomme Madrilene, ready to serve: 1 can/Crosse & Blackwell	½
Crab, ready to serve: ½ can/Crosse & Blackwell	½
Escarole, in chicken broth, ready to serve: 1 cup/Progresso	½
Gazpacho, ready to serve: ½ can/Crosse & Blackwell	½
Lentil, with ham, ready to serve: ½ can/Crosse & Blackwell	½
Lentil, ready to serve: 1 cup/Progresso	1
Meatball Alphabet, condensed, prepared: 10 oz./Campbell	2
Minestrone:	
Condensed, prepared: 10 oz./Campbell	1
Ready to Serve: ½ can (9½ oz.)/Campbell Chunky	1½
Ready to Serve: ½ can/Crosse & Blackwell	½
Mushroom:	
Condensed, prepared: 10 oz./Campbell	2
Bisque, ready to serve: ½ can/Crosse & Blackwell	2
Mix, prepared: 1 envelope/Souptime	1½
Barley, condensed, prepared: 8 oz./Manischewitz	1½
Cream of, condensed, prepared: 10 oz./Campbell	4
Cream of, semi-condensed, prepared: 1 can (11¼ oz.)/ Campbell Soup for One	4
Cream of, mix, prepared: 6 fl. oz./Lipton Cup-A-Soup	1
Noodle:	
Mix, prepared: 6 fl. oz./Lipton	½
With Beef Flavor, mix, prepared: 6 fl. oz./Lipton Cup-A-Soup	½
With Chicken, condensed, prepared: 10 oz./Campbell Curly	1
With Chicken Broth, mix, prepared: 8 fl. oz./Lipton Noodle	½
With Ground Beef, condensed, prepared: 10 oz./Campbell	2
Onion:	
Condensed, prepared: 10 oz./Campbell	1
Mix, prepared: 8 fl. oz./Lipton	½
Cream of, condensed, prepared: 10 oz./Campbell	3
Mushroom, mix, prepared: 8 fl. oz./Lipton	½
French, mix, prepared: 1 envelope/Souptime	0
Oriental Style, mix, prepared: 8 oz./Lipton Lite-Lunch	2½
Oyster Stew, condensed, prepared: 10 oz./Campbell	2
Pea, Green:	
Condensed, prepared: 10 oz./Campbell	1½
Mix, prepared: 8 fl. oz./Lipton	½
Mix, prepared: 1 envelope/Souptime	½
Pea, split, with ham, ready to serve: ½ can (9½ oz.)/Campbell Chunky	2
Pea, split, condensed, prepared: 8 oz./Manischewitz	2
Pea, split, with ham and bacon, condensed, prepared: 10 oz./Campbell	2
Pepper Pot, condensed, prepared: 10 oz./Campbell	2
Potato, cream of, condensed, prepared: 10 oz./Campbell	1

	Fat Units
Schav, condensed, prepared: 8 oz./Manischewitz	0
Scotch Broth, condensed, prepared: 10 oz./Campbell	1½
Shrimp, cream of, condensed, prepared: 10 oz./Campbell	3
Shrimp, cream, ready to serve: ½ can/Crosse & Blackwell	1½
Sirloin Burger, ready to serve: ½ can (9½ oz.)/Campbell Chunky	3
Steak & Potato, ready to serve: ½ can (9½ oz.)/Campbell Chunky	2
Stockpot, vegetable, mix, prepared: 8 oz./Lipton Lite-Lunch	3
Stockpot, vegetable-beef, condensed, prepared: 10 oz./Campbell	2
Tomato:	
Condensed, prepared: 10 oz./Campbell	½
Condensed, prepared: 8 oz./Manischewitz	1½
Ready to Serve: 8 fl. oz./Progresso	½
Mix, prepared: 6 fl. oz./Lipton Cup-A-Soup	½
Mix, prepared: 1 envelope/Souptime	½
Beef, condensed, prepared: 10 oz./Campbell NoodleO's	2
Bisque, condensed, prepared: 10 oz./Campbell	1
Rice, condensed, prepared: 10 oz./Campbell Old Fashioned	½
Turkey:	
Ready to Serve: ½ can (9¼ oz.)/Campbell Chunky	2
Noodle, condensed, prepared: 10 oz./Campbell	1
Vegetable, condensed, prepared: 10 oz./Campbell	1½
Vegetable:	
Condensed, prepared: 10 oz./Campbell	½
Condensed, prepared: 10 oz./Campbell Old Fashioned	1½
Canned, ready to serve, individual service size: 1 can (10¾ oz.)/ Campbell Chunky	1½
Condensed, prepared: 8 oz./Manischewitz	1
Semi-Condensed, prepared: 1 can/Campbell Old World Soup for One	1½
Mix, prepared: 8 fl. oz./Lipton Country	½
Beef, condensed, prepared: 10 oz./Campbell	1
Beef, ready to serve: ½ can (9½ oz.)/Campbell Chunky	2
Beef, mix, prepared: 8 fl. oz./Lipton	½
Beef, mix, prepared: 6 fl. oz./Lipton Cup-A-Soup	½
Beef, with shells, mix, prepared: 8 fl. oz./Lipton	½
Cream of, mix prepared: 1 envelope/Souptime	1½
With Noodles, condensed, prepared: 10 oz./Campbell NoodleO's	1
Vichyssoise, ready to serve: ½ can/Crosse & Blackwell	1½

SPAGHETTI DISHES

Spaghetti in tomato sauce, canned:	
Buitoni TWISTS: ½ can	1
With Cheese: 7⅜ oz./Franco-American	1
With Cheese Sauce: 7⅜ oz./Franco-American "SpaghettiOs"	1
With Frankfurters: 7⅜ oz./Franco-American "SpaghettiOs"	3½
With Meat Sauce: 7¾ oz./Franco American	3½
With Meatballs: ½ can/Buitoni	3
With Little Meatballs: 7⅜ oz./Franco-American "SpaghettiOs"	3
Spaghetti with sauce, frozen:	
Banquet: 3 oz.	5
Morton Casserole: 1 pkg	2
Stouffer: 1 pkg, 14 oz.	4

	Fat Units
With Meatballs 9 oz./Green Giant Boil-in-Bag Entrees	4
Spaghetti and Sauce, mixes:	
Prepared: 1 pouch/Betty Crocker Mug-O-Lunch	1
Prepared: 1 cup/Kraft Tangy Italian Style	2

STUFFING MIXES

Chicken & Herb: 1 oz./Pepperidge Farm Pan Style	½
Chicken-Flavored, prepared with butter: ½ cup/Stove Top	3
Chicken-Flavored, prepared: ½ cup cooked with butter/Uncle Ben's	
Stuff'n Such	3½
½ cup cooked without butter/Uncle Ben's Stuff'n Such	½
Corn Bread: 1 oz. dry/Pepperidge Farm	½
Cornbread, prepared with butter: ½ cup/Stove Top	3
Corn Bread, prepared: ½ cup cooked with butter/Uncle Ben's	
Stuff'n Such	3½
½ cup cooked without butter	½
Cube: 1 oz. dry/Pepperidge Farm	½
Sage: ½ cup cooked with butter/Uncle Ben's Stuff'n Such	3½
½ cup cooked without butter	½
Pork-Flavored, mix, prepared with butter: ½ cup/Stove Top	3
With Rice, prepared with butter: ½ cup/Stove Top	3

TOASTER PASTRIES   1 portion

Pop Tarts: 1 tart/Kellogg's	2½

TOPPINGS

Chocolate:	
Smucker's/1 tbsp	½
Fudge: 1 tbsp/Hershey's	½
Pecans in Syrup: 1 tbsp/Smucker's	½
Peanut Butter Caramel: 1 tbsp/Smucker's	½
Pineapple: 1 tbsp/Smucker's	½
Strawberry: 1 tbsp/Smucker's	½
Walnuts in Syrup: 1 tbsp/Smucker's	½
Whipped, nondairy, frozen: 1 tbsp/Cool Whip	½
Whipped, mix, prepared: 1 tbsp/Dream Whip	½
Whipped, mix, prepared: 1 tbsp/D-Zerta	½
No-Cal, various flavors: 1 tbsp	0

VEGETABLES   ⅓ pkg = about ½ cup

Canned and Frozen:	
Asparagus/all brands	0
Beans, baked: 1 cup/B & M	3
Beans, baked style:	
With Bacon: 7½ oz. can/Hormel Short Orders	4
In Barbecue Sauce: 8 oz./Campbell	2
With Frankfurters: 7½ oz. can/Hormel Short Orders Beans 'n Wieners	5

	Fat Units
With Frankfurters, in tomato and molasses sauce: 8 oz. Campbell Beans and Franks	5½
With Ham: 7½ oz. can/Hormel Short Orders	6½
In Molasses and Brown Sugar Sauce: 8 oz./Campbell Old Fashioned	2
With Pork, in tomato sauce: 8 oz./Campbell	1½
Beans, black turtle, canned: 1 cup/Progresso	½
Beans, fava, canned: 1 cup/Progresso	½
Beans, green, canned or frozen, plain/all brands	0
Beans, green, frozen:	
Cut, in butter sauce: 1 cup/Green Giant	1½
French, in butter sauce: 1 cup/Green Giant	1½
French, with sliced mushrooms: Birds Eye	0
French, with toasted almonds: 3 oz. (about ½ cup)/Birds Eye	½
With Onions and Bacon Bits: 1 cup/Green Giant	1½
And Pearl Onions, 3 oz. (about ½ cup)/Birds Eye	0
And Spaetzle, with sauce: 3.3 oz. (about ½ cup)/Birds Eye	½
Beans, kidney, red: 1 cup/Progresso	½
Beans, lima:	
Plain: 1 cup/all brands	½
Baby, in butter sauce, frozen: 1 cup/Green Giant	2
Beans, pinto, canned: 1 cup/Progresso	½
Beans, salad, canned: 1 cup/Green Giant 3-Bean	½
Beans, wax or yellow/all brands	0
Beets/all brands	0
Broccoli, frozen:	
Plain/all brands	0
Au Gratin: ½ pkg/Stouffer	4
With Cauliflower and Carrots, in cheese sauce: 1 cup/Green Giant	2
With Cheese Sauce: 3.3 oz. (about ½ cup)/Birds Eye	3
With Cheese Sauce: 1 cup/Green Giant	2
With Cheese Sauce: 1 cup/Green Giant Bake 'n Serve	6½
Spears, in butter sauce: 1 cup/Green Giant	2
Brussels Sprouts, frozen:	
Plain/all brands	0
In Butter Sauce: 1 cup/Green Giant	2
Halves 'n Cheese Sauce: 1 cup/Green Giant	2½
Butterbeans, canned: 8 oz./Sultana	½
Butterbeans, speckled, frozen: 1 cup/Green Giant Southern Recipe	4
Carrots:	
Plain/all brands	0
With Brown Sugar Glaze, frozen: 3.3 oz./Birds Eye	½
In Butter Sauce, frozen: 1 cup/Green Giant Nuggets	2
Cauliflower, frozen:	
Plain/all brands	0
With Cheese Sauce: 3.3 oz./Birds Eye	2½
In Cheese Sauce: 1 cup/Green Giant	2
In Cheese Sauce: 1 cup/Green Giant Bake 'n Serve	5½
Chick Peas, canned: 1 cup/Progresso	1
Collard Greens, frozen/all brands	0
Corn, canned: 1 cup/all brands	½
With Peppers: 1 cup/Del Monte Corn 'n Peppers	½
With Peppers: 1 cup/Green Giant Mexicorn	½

	Fat Units
Corn, golden, frozen:	
In Butter Sauce: 1 cup/Green Giant Niblets	2
On Cob: 1 ear/Birds Eye	½
On Cob: 1 ear/Green Giant	½
With Peppers in Butter Sauce: 1 cup/Green Giant Mexican	2
Soufflé: ⅓ pkg/Stouffer	2½
Corn, white: in butter sauce, frozen: 1 cup/Green Giant	2
Eggplant Parmesan, frozen: 5½ oz./Mrs. Paul's	5½
Eggplant Sticks, fried, frozen: 3½ oz./Mrs. Paul's	5½
Eggplant Slices, fried, frozen: 3 oz./Mrs. Paul's	5½
Green Peppers, stuffed, frozen: 1 pkg/Stouffer	4
Kale, frozen/all brands	0
Mixed, frozen:	
Cantonese style: 3.3 oz./Birds Eye Stir Fry	0
Chinese: 1 pkg/La Choy	½
Chinese: 1 cup/Green Giant	1½
Chinese, witth sauce: 3.3 oz./Birds Eye International	0
Chinese, with seasonings: 3.3 oz./Birds Eye Stir Fry	0
Danish Style, with sauce: 3.3 oz./Birds Eye International	0
Hawaiian Style: 1 cup/Green Giant Boil-in-Bag	2½
Hawaiian Style: 3.3 oz./Birds Eye	0
Italian Style with Sauce: 3.3 oz/Birds Eye	½
Japanese: 1 pkg/La Choy	0
Japanese Style: 1 cup/Green Giant Boil-in-Bag	1
Japanese Style, with sauce: 3.3 oz./Birds Eye International	0
Japanese Style, with seasonings: 3.3 oz./Birds Eye Stir Fry	0
Jubilee: 3.3 oz./Birds Eye Combinations	2
Mandarin Style with Seasonings: 3.3 oz./Birds Eye Stir Fry	0
New England Style: 3.3 oz./Birds Eye Americana Recipe	½
New Orleans Creole Style: 3.3 oz./Birds Eye Americana Recipe	0
Parisian Style with Sauce: 3.3 oz./Birds Eye International	0
Pennsylvania Dutch Style: 3.3 oz./Birds Eye Americana Recipe	½
San Francisco Style: 3.3 oz./Birds Eye Americana Recipe	½
Wisconsin Country Style: 3.3 oz./Birds Eye Americana Recipe	½
In Butter Sauce: 1 cup/Green Giant	2
In Onion Sauce: 2.6 oz./Birds Eye	2
Mushrooms, plain/all brands	0
Mushrooms, in butter sauce, frozen: 2 oz./Green Giant	½
Okra Gumbo, frozen: 1 cup/Green Giant Boil-in-Bag Southern Recipe	6½
Onions, frozen:	
In Cheese-Flavor Sauce: 1 cup/Green Giant	3
In Cream Sauce: 3 oz./Birds Eye	2
Onion Rings, fried, canned: 1 oz./O & C	5½
Onion Rings, fried, frozen: 2½ oz./Mrs. Paul's	2½
Onion Rings, fried, frozen: 2 oz./Ore-Ida Onion Ringers	4
Peas, black-eye:	
Canned: 1 cup/Progresso	½
Canned with Pork: 8 oz./Sultana	1½
Frozen: 3.3 oz./Birds Eye	0
Frozen: 1 cup/Green Giant Boil-in-Bag Southern Recipe	4
Peas, green, canned: plain/all brands	0

	Fat Units
Peas, green, frozen:	
Plain/all brands	0
In Butter Sauce: 1 cup/Green Giant	2
And Cauliflower with Cream Sauce: 3.3 oz./Birds Eye Combinations	2
With Cream Sauce: 2.6 oz./Birds Eye Combinations	2½
Creamed with Bread Crumb Topping: 1 cup/Green Giant Bake n' Serve	5½
With Onions and Carrots in Butter Sauce: 1 cup/Le Sueur	2
With Pea Pods and Water Chestnuts in Sauce: 1 cup/Le Sueur	3
And Pearl Onions: 3.3 oz./Birds Eye Combinations	0
And Potatoes with Cream Sauce: 2.6 oz./Birds Eye Combinations	2½
With Sliced Mushrooms: 3.3 oz./Birds Eye Combinations	0
Potatoes, frozen:	
Au Gratin: 1 cup/Green Giant Bake 'n Serve	9
Au Gratin: ⅓ pkg/Stouffer	3
Diced, in sour cream sauce: 1 cup/Green Giant Boil-in-Bag	4
French Fried: 2.8 oz./Birds Eye Cottage Fries	2
French Fried: 3 oz./Birds Eye	1½
French Fried: 3 oz./Ore-Ida Cottage Fries	2
French Fried: 3 oz./Ore-Ida Crispers	5½
French Fried: 3 oz./Ore-Ida Self Sizzling Fries	3
French Fried: 3 oz./Ore-Ida Self Sizzling Shoestrings	4
Fried: 3 oz./Birds Eye Deep Gold	2
Fried: 2.5 oz./Birds Eye Tasti Puffs	4
Fried: 3.2 oz./Birds Eye Tiny Taters	4
Hash Browns: 4 oz./Birds Eye	½
Hash Browns with Butter Sauce: 3 oz./Ore-Ida Southern Style	2
Hash Browns with Butter Sauce and Onions: 3 oz./Ore-Ida Southern Style	3
Scalloped: ⅓ pkg/Stouffer	2½
Slices in Butter Sauce: 1 cup/Green Giant Boil-in-Bag	3½
Slices in Butter Sauce: 1 cup/Green Giant Boil-in-Bag	3½
Stuffed with Cheese-Flavored Topping: 5 oz./Green Giant Oven Bake	4
Stuffed with Sour Cream and Chives: 5 oz./Green Giant Oven Bake	3½
Shoestring in Butter Sauce: 1 cup/Green Giant Boil-in-Bag	6
And Sweet Peas in Bacon Cream Sauce: 1 cup/Green Giant Boil-in-Bag	3½
Tater Tots: 3 oz./Ore-Ida	2½
Vermicelli: 1 cup/Green Giant Bake 'n Serve	7
Potatoes, mix, prepared:	
Au Gratin: ½ cup/Betty Crocker	2
Au Gratin: ½ cup/French's Big Tate	2
Creamed: ½ cup/Betty Crocker	2½
Hash Brown: ½ cup/French's Big Tate	3
Hash Brown with Onions: ½ cup/Betty Crocker	2
Potato Buds: ½ cup/Betty Crocker	2
Mashed: ½ cup/French's	2
Mashed: ½ cup/French's Big Tate	2½
Mashed: ½ cup/Hungry Jack (4 serving container)	3½
Pancakes: three 3-in. cakes/French's Big Tate	2
Scalloped: ½ cup/Betty Crocker	2

	Fat Units
Potatoes, sweet, frozen:	
Glazed: 1 cup/Green Giant Boil-in-Bag Southern Recipe	3
Candied: 4 oz./Mrs. Paul's	2
Candied with Apples: 4 oz./Mrs. Paul's	2
Candied, orange: 4 oz./Mrs. Paul's	2
Pumpkin, canned: 1 cup/Del Monte	½
Sauerkraut, canned/all brands	0
Soup Greens, in jar: 1 jar/Durkee	1
Spinach, canned and frozen:	
Plain/all brands	0
In Butter Sauce: 1 cup/Green Giant	2
Creamed: 3 oz./Birds Eye Combinations	1½
Creamed: 1 cup/Green Giant	3
Soufflé: 1 cup/Green Giant Bake 'n Serve	6
Soufflé ⅓ pkg/Stouffer	2½
Squash, cooked, frozen: 4 oz./Birds Eye	0
Squash, summer in cheese sauce, frozen: 1 cup/Green Giant Boil-in-Bag	1½
Stew, vegetable, canned: 7½ oz./Dinty Moore	3
Stew, vegetable, frozen: 3 oz./Ore-Ida	0
Succotash, canned: 1 cup/Stokely-Van Camp	½
Tomato Paste, canned/all brands	0
Tomatoes, canned/all brands	0
Turnip Greens, canned or frozen/all brands	0
Zucchini, sticks, in light batter: 3 oz./Mrs. Paul's	3
Zucchini, in tomato sauce, canned: 1 cup/Del Monte	0

YOGURT, FROZEN

Danny Flip/5 fl. oz.	1½
Danny Parfait/4 fl. oz.	1½
Danny Sampler/3 fl. oz.	½
Danny-Yo/3½ fl. oz.	1½
Danny In-A-Cup, plain and fruit/8 fl. oz.	2
Peach: ½ cup/Sealtest	1
Red Raspberry: ½ cup/Sealtest	1
Vanilla: ½ cup/Sealtest	1
Bars:	
Carob-Coated: 1 bar/Danny On A Stick	2½
Chocolate-Coated: 1 bar/Danny On-A-Stick	2½
Uncoated: 1 bar/Danny On-A-Stick	½
Yosicle/2½ fl. oz.	½

FAST FOODS

	Fat Units
ARBY's	
Roast Beef Sandwich	5½
Beef and Cheese Sandwich	8
Super Roast Beef Sandwich	10
Junior Roast Beef Sandwich	3
Swiss King Sandwich	12
Ham 'N Cheese Sandwich	6
Turkey Sandwich	6½
Turkey Deluxe Sandwich	8½
Club Sandwich	10½
ARTHUR TREACHER'S	
Fish—two pieces	4½
Chicken—two pieces	5½
Shrimp—7 pieces	7½
Chips	4
Krunch Pup	9
Cole Slaw	3
Lemon Luvs	5½
Chowder	1
Fish Sandwich	5½
Chicken Sandwich	4
BURGER CHEF	
Hamburger	4½
Cheeseburger	6
Double Cheeseburger	9
Big Shef	12
Super Shef	13
Skipper's Treat	13
French Fries	3
Shakes	4
Mariner Platter	8½
Rancher Platter	13½
BURGER KING	
Whopper	13
Double Beef Whopper	18½
Whopper with Cheese	16
Double Beef Whopper with Cheese	21½
Whopper Junior	7
Whopper Junior with Cheese	8½
Whopper Jr. with Double Meat	10
Whopper Jr. Double Meat Pattie with Cheese	12

	Fat Units
Hamburger	5
Hamburger with Cheese	6½
Double Meat Hamburger	8
Double Meat Hamburger with Cheese	11½
Steak Sandwich	7½
Whaler	13
Whaler with Cheese	16
Onion Rings—Large	6½
Onion Rings—Regular	4½
French Fries—Large Bag	6½
French Fries—Regular Bag	4
Chocolate or Vanilla Milkshake	4
Apple Pie	4

CHURCH'S FRIED CHICKEN

1 average piece boned dark	7½
1 average piece boned white	8

DAIRY QUEEN/BRAZIER

Snacks and Desserts	
Cone—Regular	2½
Chocolate Dipped Cone—Regular	4½
Chocolate Sundae—Regular	2½
Chocolate Malt—Regular	7
Float	3
Banana Split	5½
Parfait	4
"Fiesta" Sundae	8
Freeze	4½
"Mr. Misty" Freeze	4
"Mr. Misty" Float	3
"Dilly" Bar	5½
"DQ" Sandwich	1½
"Mr. Misty" Kiss	½
Hamburger	3½
Cheeseburger	5
Big "Brazier"	8
Big "Brazier" with Cheese	10½
Super "Brazier"/The "Half Pounder"	17
Hot Dog	5½
Hot Dog with Chili	7
Hot Dog with Cheese	6½
Fish Sandwich	6
Fish Sandwich with Cheese	7½
French Fries	3½
Onion Rings	6

HARDEE'S

Hamburger	5½
Cheeseburger	5½

	Fat Units
Huskie	14½
Big Twin	9
French Fries—Small	4½
French Fries—Large	7½
Apple Turnover	5
Milkshake	3½
Roast Beef Sandwich	5½
Fish Sandwich	9
Hot Dog	8

KENTUCKY FRIED CHICKEN

Chicken Dinner: 3 pieces chicken with mashed potatoes and gravy, cole slaw, and roll	
KFC Original Recipe Dinner	16
KFC Extra-Crispy Dinner	19
Individual pieces, Original Recipe:	
Wing	3½
Drumstick	3
Breast	4½
Rib	5
Thigh	6½

LONG JOHN SILVER'S SEAFOOD SHOPPES

Fish with Batter (2 pc. order)	8½
Treasure Chest (1 pc. fish & 3 peg legs)	10
Chicken Planks (4 pc. order)	8
Peg Legs with Batter (5 pc. order)	11½
Ocean Scallops (6 pc. order)	4
Shrimp with Batter (6 pc. avg. order)	4½
Breaded Oysters	6½
Breaded Clams	9
S.O.S. Super Ocean Sandwich	10½
Fryes	5½
Cole Slaw	3
Corn on the Cob	1½
Hush Puppies	2½

McDONALD'S

Hamburger	3½
Cheeseburger	4½
Quarter Pounder	7
Quarter Pounder with Cheese	10
Big Mac	11
Filet-O-Fish	8
Egg McMuffin	7
Hot Cakes with Butter and Syrup	3
Scrambled Eggs	4
Pork Sausage	6
English Muffin (Buttered)	2

	Fat Units
French Fries	4
Apple Pie	6½
Cherry Pie	6½
McDonaldland Cookies	4
Chocolate Shake	3
Vanilla Shake	3
Strawberry Shake	3

PIZZA HUT

Serving size: one-half of a 10-inch pizza (3 slices)	
Thin 'N Crispy Pizza:	
Beef	6½
Pork	8
Cheese	5½
Pepperoni	6
Supreme	7½
Thick 'N Chewy Pizza:	
Beef	7
Pork	8
Cheese	5
Pepperoni	6½
Supreme	8

TACO BELL

Bean Burrito	4
Beef Burrito	7½
Beefy Tostada	5½
Bellbeefer	2½
Bellbeefer with Cheese	4
Burrito Supreme	8
Combination Burrito	5½
Enchirito	7½
Pintos 'N Cheese	2
Taco	3
Tostada	2

AFTERWORD:

An Important Message

THE CASE AGAINST FAT

Americans on the average now eat over 40 percent of their calories daily in fat. That's not extraordinary when compared with European or Scandinavian countries, where dairy products are common. All so-called Western diets are high in fat. In comparison, many Oriental and African diets where grain is the main staple, instead of meats and dairy products, are low in fats. The pre-World War II Japanese, subsisting on rice and fish, ate about 10 percent of their calories in fat. But with the influence of the Western world, the Japanese diet has been changing and going up in fat. So, too, has the incidence of Western-type diseases, mainly heart disease and cancer.

The consumption of fat in the U.S. has been rising since the turn of the century. The number of calories we consume daily has barely changed since 1910, nor has the proportion of calories that comes from protein. But, the amount of those calories that come from *fat* has gone up 25 percent. And the number of calories attributed to carbohydrates (except sugar) has dropped by an equal percentage. In other words, we have almost directly replaced our complex carbohydrates, notably grains, with fat.

You're eating on the average about 2½ tablespoons more fat today than an American at the turn of the century—or 24 pounds more fat a year. Most of that rise is attributed to salad and cooking oils; however, recently meat, namely beef, has become the primary contributor to the rise in fat intake.

Health specialists almost unanimously agree that most people are eating too much fat. Some say we should not eat more than one-third or 30 percent of our calories in fat. For example, Senator George McGovern's nutrition subcommittee in its well-publicized "dietary goals" recommended reducing the fat intake to one-third of calories and replacing it with grains, fruits, and vegetables.

Reprinted from THE ALL-IN-ONE LOW FAT GRAM COUNTER by Jean Carper, Bantam Books, Inc., 1980. By permission of the author.

Nathan Pritikin and an increasing number of other health experts are recommending cutting down on all kinds of fat—saturated, or animal, fats as well as unsaturated, or vegetable, fats. They believe that excessive amounts of either or both are dangerous to your health.

FAT AND HEART DISEASE

A high fat diet can contribute to heart disease in two ways—directly and indirectly. One way is by putting saturated fats into the body, which raises the blood cholesterol believed to lead to atherosclerosis and heart disease. And the second way is by replacing the complex carbohydrates in the diet that may lower cholesterol, protecting against heart disease. Studies show that when people cut down on fat in the diet, they automatically eat more carbohydrates, such as whole grains and vegetables.

Countless studies have been done both on animals and humans showing that high blood cholesterol levels are related to heart disease and that the cholesterol can be lowered through a low saturated fat, low cholesterol diet. At least fifteen expert committees on dietary fat and heart disease have recommended lowering the intake of the percentage of calories derived from fat to between 25 and 35 percent. After a comprehensive study of the literature on diet and heart disease, Dr. Jeremiah Stamler, writing in the medical journal *Circulation,* July 1978, concluded: "It is reasonable and sound to designate 'rich' (high-fat) diet as a primary, essential, necessary cause of the current epidemic of premature atherosclerotic disease raging in the Western industrialized countries."

Generally cholesterol is blamed as the main culprit. Thus, some people will cut down on high cholesterol foods such as shrimp and eggs and still go on eating high fat foods such as beef and coconut. What they don't realize is that these saturated, high-fat foods also raise cholesterol levels in the blood—even more so than high-cholesterol foods do. Patricia Hausman, a nutritionist at the Center for Science in the Public Interest, a Washington, D.C., based public interest group specializing in health and nutrition, points out that just because foods are low in cholesterol does not necessarily mean they are all right for your arteries.

Yet, meat and dairy producers sometimes tout their products as low in cholesterol, never mentioning they are high in fat. Here is a quote from a flyer from the National Livestock and Meat Board: "Steaks, chops and roasts are not full of cholesterol as many have come to believe. . . . Many people are adjusting their diets to control cholesterol by eating less meat and butter, fewer eggs and more poultry and fish. Yet, according to the Meat Board, meat is lower in cholesterol than a number of poultry, fish and seafood items."

The Dairy Council publicizes that milk and other dairy products are not high in cholesterol. And the candy bar makers will tell you that chocolate is not high in cholesterol. It is true, of course, but it can be misleading. For although meat, milk, cheese, and chocolate may not be high in cholesterol, they are high in saturated fats that can raise cholesterol levels in the blood.

Ms. Hausman writes: "Talking only about the cholesterol in foods and not mentioning saturated fat is a common tactic of the meat and dairy industries. The public associates cholesterol in food with cholesterol in the blood, well aware that the higher their blood cholesterol levels, the greater the risk of heart disease and in some cases, stroke. But fewer people know that saturated fat also increases their blood cholesterol—even more so than the cholesterol in foods. The dairy and meat industries try to hide this fact because high-fat dairy products and many meats have a hefty share of saturated fat."

Hausman says that although shrimp is exceptionally high in cholesterol, it actually raises the cholesterol in your blood to about the same extent as a piece of lean meat that has only moderate amounts of cholesterol. The high fat content of the meat does the trick.

Thus, if you want to cut down on true blood cholesterol levels, you must also curtail your intake of highly saturated fats.

Further, replacing fatty foods with carbohydrates may have a protective effect against heart disease. Studies show that those with a low incidence of coronary heart disease—mainly vegetarians—consume from 65 to 85 percent of their diet in carbohydrates from whole grains (mainly cereals) and vegetables (mainly potatoes).

Dr. Stamler also points out that Southern Italians, who have a starchy diet (about 40 to 55 percent of their calories from carbohydrates), have lower blood cholesterol levels.

Although heart specialists for years have condemned saturated fats, there is increasing evidence that unsaturated fats too may be more detrimental than previously believed. Pritikin claims that "all excess fats are bad for you, animal and vegetable, saturated and unsaturated." For one reason, he says, because fats of all kinds have a suffocating effect on the blood. He says eating too much fat encloses part of the blood in a fatty film, causing clumps to form that plug up small blood vessels, resulting in a shutdown of from 5 to 20 percent of your blood circulation. He also says unsaturated fats such as vegetable oils can boost the levels of triglycerides—fatty acids also linked to heart disease.

Although the conventional wisdom in recent years has been to substitute unsaturated fats, such as margarine, for saturated fats, such as butter, to prevent heart disease, some new questions are being raised about the safety of margarine. Some studies suggest that when margarine is hydrogenated (hardened) it forms new molecular structures that could be detrimental to the body. Dr. Hugh Sinclair, at the Laboratory of Human Nutrition at Oxford University in England, found that hydrogenated fats caused a deficiency of essential fatty acids in the bodies of both animals and humans. He said such a deficiency "contributed to neurological diseases, heart disease, arteriosclerosis, skin disease, various degenerative conditions such as cataract and arthritis and cancer."

At the University of Illinois, food chemistry professor Fred Kummerow fed pigs hydrogenated fat containing high amounts of trans fatty acids and found that 58 percent of them developed early signs of atherosclerosis. That was compared with only 14 percent for those not fed the hydrogenated fat. Interestingly, the animals fed the hydrogenated fat had higher levels of cholesterol in the blood.

Recently, a scientist in Israel, Professor S. Hillel Blondheim, found evidence, after a two-year study, contradicting the traditional views of heart disease and diet. He found that a group of Bedouin who had become Westernized and ate more unsaturated fats had a higher level of blood cholesterol than tribesmen who ate saturated fats. Said Professor Blondheim: "Here's a population among whom incidence of heart disease was nil, although all the fat in the traditional diet was of animal origin. Now those in steady contact with Westernized culture appear to be consuming more polyunsaturates; and yet, as far as we can tell from the limited number of cases in our sample, they are precisely the ones who have higher levels of serum cholesterol. This might knock the accepted theories into a cocked hat."

Obviously, not everything is known about the effects of fats of all kinds on heart disease, but there is sufficient evidence to show that it is detrimental and that perhaps the safest course of all, as some scientists recommend, is to cut down on the consumption of all kinds of fat—saturated and unsaturated, animal and vegetable.

FAT AND CANCER

There's also increasing evidence that fats of all kinds, both animal and vegetable, may be related to cancer. The evidence is not conclusive, but it is compelling enough that the National Cancer Institute recently recommended reducing the fat content in the diet to one-third of the calories as a possible way of preventing cancer.

The theory has been promoted vigorously by Dr. Ernst Wynder, head of the American Health Foundation and a prominent cancer researcher. Dr. Wynder in 1965 presented a paper showing a worldwide correlation between eating high amounts of animal fat and high rates of colon cancer. He said this pattern, tying colon cancer to the "high-fat Western diet," was clear in this country, the Netherlands, Belgium, Denmark, West Germany, France, England and Canada. In contrast, he noted that the Japanese, who at the time ate one-fourth as much animal fat as we do, had a colon cancer rate of only 2.5 per 100,000 compared with 14 per 100,000 in the United States.

Further, the Japanese who move to this country develop higher rates of cancer. The reasonable explanation, says Dr. Wynder, is a change in the diet. Also, animal studies dating back to the 1930s and 1940s show that animals exposed to cancer-causing chemicals develop more cancers when they are fed high fat diets.

The theory lately has gathered more advocates. And a high fat diet has now been linked by many studies to several kinds of cancer: notably breast, but also cancer of the prostate, pancreas, ovaries, kidney and bladder.

At first Dr. Wynder and others believed that cancer was associated only with animal, or saturated, fats. But lately that theory has been turned topsy-turvy. Recent, well-respected tests show that vegetable, or unsaturated, fats may be even a more potent cancer producer than animal fats. Kenneth Carroll, a biochemist at the University of Ontario, showed that when you feed carcinogen-exposed rats high amounts of unsaturated fats—such as olive, corn and safflower oil—they develop twice as many tumors as rats exclusively fed saturated fats such as butter and meat fat.

What's more, when you mix only small amounts of unsaturated fats (3 percent of the diet) with saturated fats, you get even more cancer in rats than you would with either alone. The unsaturated fats somehow potentiate the cancer production.

Nobody at this point knows why this happens, but Carroll and other experts, in the absence of more precise knowledge, advise that everyone should severely reduce their fat intake—of all kinds—as a precaution against cancer. At the moment, many cancer scientists are advising cutting back to at least 30 percent of calories from fat —the same amount generally recommended by heart specialists. However, this may not be enough to prevent cancer.

Dr. John Weisburger, a well-known cancer researcher working at the American Health Foundation with Dr. Wynder, points out we may have to reduce our fat intake even further—perhaps to 20 or even 10 percent of calories. He notes that prior to World War II, the Japanese, when they had an exceptionally low rate of cancer, were eating only 10 percent of their calories in fat. This is along the lines recommended by the Pritikin diet. Dr. Weisburger notes that studies on animals in England have shown that animals who ate 30 percent of their calories in fat had just as high a rate of cancer as those who ate 60 percent of their calories in fat. So, he suggests, the cutback to 30 percent may not be severe enough to prevent cancer;

more studies, he says, are needed to define more precisely the permissible amount of fat.

However, there's another avenue of benefit. At the same time you reduce your fat content, you will eat more vegetables and grain, and they in themselves may protect you from cancer. There is evidence that a higher consumption of grains and fruits and vegetables will reduce the chances of cancer. One theory is that fiber in grain (cereals and whole-grain breads) protects against cancer; thus, the National Cancer Institute also recommends increasing fiber as you cut fat. Another theory is that the vegetables themselves contain specific chemicals that counteract the effects of cancer. This is not as off-the-wall as it may sound at first.

Dr. Saxon Graham, at the State University of New York at Buffalo, found that people who ate the most cabbage—yes, plain old cabbage, whether cooked or raw, as sauerkraut or cole slaw—were less likely to have colon cancer. Further, a chemical has been isolated from such vegetables that does prevent cancer in laboratory animals. Professor Lee Wattenberg at the University of Minnesota found that a chemical called "indoles" reduces the rate of cancer in animals exposed to cancer-causing substances. Dr. Wattenberg exposed animals to carcinogenic substances and at the same time gave some of them indoles. In one test 81 percent of the rats who did *not* get indoles developed breast cancer. But only 21 to 27 percent of the rats given indoles as an antidote developed breast cancer.

The important point is that these indoles are found naturally in certain vegetables, including cabbage. Other vegetables that also have indoles are Brussels sprouts, turnips, cauliflower and broccoli. Perhaps it's not surprising then that vegetarians often have a lower cancer rate than meat eaters.

How a high fat diet might produce cancer is unknown. But scientists, including Dr. Wynder, believe fat is not a direct initiator of cancer (in the way pesticides are). Instead, they believe it is a "cancer promoter." In other words, eating fat somehow encourages the cancer to grow. It might do this, Wynder theorizes, by causing the body through complicated mechanisms to produce substances that promote cancer growth. For example, according to Dr. Wynder, excessive fat produces high amounts of bile acids in the colon, and bile acids have produced cancer in laboratory animals. Also, studies show that colon cancer victims often have higher concentrations of bile acids.

As for breast cancer, the theory is that a high fat diet encourages a disproportionate production of a hormone called prolactin. Prolactin has been proved as a cancer promoter in animals. Further, Wynder has shown that women who go on low fat vegetarian diets produce less prolactin than when they're eating high fat meats.

Although all the evidence is not in, many believe it is sufficiently persuasive to encourage people to reduce their fat intake to prevent cancer. Dr. Wynder strongly believes that women who already have breast cancer should cut down on fatty foods to slow the growth of cancer. Even if the evidence is not firm, many scientists say cutting down on fat certainly can't hurt you, and it will do your general health and weight a lot of good.

FAT AND OTHER HEALTH PROBLEMS

One of the greatest dangers of overdosing on fatty foods is getting fat yourself. It is very difficult to continue day after day on a high fat diet and control your weight. Studies show that people with severe weight problems usually consume high quantities of fatty foods.

Not only is overweight a problem in itself, it leads to other health problems. Dr. Theodore Cooper, former assistant secretary for health, has said: "Overweight aggravates cardiovascular disease and osteoarthritis, and increases the liability to hypertension, atherosclerosis, hernia and gall bladder disease. It may also facilitate the emergence of latent diabetes in predisposed individuals as they approach an advanced age and adds to the hazards of surgery. . . . Statistics make it quite clear that the obese do not live as long as the lean. The chief cause of death among overweight individuals is cardiovascular-renal diseases, diabetes and disorders of the liver and biliary tract (the gallbladder)."

Additionally, fatty foods are often not very nutritious; and consuming them in place of better foods, such as grains and fruits and vegetables, deprives you of nutrients. Fats such as salad oils and lard provide relatively empty calories—little different in nutrient value from the calories from alcohol and sugar—that produce energy and weight gain but little else.

HOW TO TELL SATURATED FROM UNSATURATED FATS

Doctors sometimes make a distinction between "saturated" and "unsaturated" fats. Technically this is a distinction in the chemical makeup of the fatty acids. Saturated fat has a hydrogen atom attached to each of its carbon atoms in the chain; unsaturated fat has at least two carbon atoms to which no hydrogen atom is attached. However, the fatty acids in foods are not entirely saturated or unsaturated. All kinds of foods—meats, dairy products, vegetables— have varying amounts of saturated and unsaturated fats. So a food is not *exclusively* a saturated or unsaturated fatty food. A food is said to be high in saturated fat when the fat content is predominately one or the other. For example, the fat in safflower oil is 74 percent unsaturated; thus it is referred to as an unsaturated, or often a polyunsaturated, fatty food. In contrast, butter and beef fat are around 50 percent saturated fat; thus, they are called saturated fatty foods.

You will not find the fat grams in this book broken down into percentages of saturated and unsaturated fats. The premise of this book, which is consistent with much current scientific and nutritional thinking, is that it is wise to cut down on fat per se—regardless of whether it is saturated or unsaturated.

However, if you are more concerned about saturated fats, all you need to know as a rule is that saturated fats are found primarily in animal foods—meat, eggs, milk, cream, cheese. And the fat in vegetable products is mostly unsaturated. Fish, too, is low in saturated fats. The dramatic exceptions to this rule are coconut and palm oil, both highly saturated in fat content.

CHOLESTEROL CONTENT OF FOODS

Cholesterol, though technically not a fat, is a chemical component of animal fats; it is a waxy fatlike substance that does not dissolve in water or blood. The theory is that excessive cholesterol in the blood clumps and attaches itself to artery walls, leading to formation of "arterial plaque." As plaque builds up, it closes off arteries and helps cause heart attacks and strokes in some persons. Heart experts believe that the amount of cholesterol in the blood (serum cholesterol) is strongly predictive of the chances of having a heart attack—at least up until age fifty. After that other factors may be more important.

An expert study group recently convened by the American Health Foundation reported that average blood cholesterol levels among Americans are alarmingly high, even among children, and that they should be reduced by 25 percent. Although many physicians tell patients their cholesterol count is "normal" if it's no higher than 250 milligrams of cholesterol per deciliter, the study group agreed that the average level should be no more than 180 to 190. Dr. Henry Blackburn, director of the Laboratory of Physiological Hygiene at the University of Minnesota, says 150 to 160 is "ideal" to prevent heart attacks and artery disease.

Cholesterol—like fat—is *not* found in vegetable products in any significant amount. However, you may have noticed that some food companies advertise "cholesterol free" peanut-butter, and even "cholesterol free" cereals. Technically this is correct, but it has no meaning. Such advertising campaigns are meant to exploit an unknowledgable public.

Remember:

- You don't have to worry about vegetable products having cholesterol, regardless of the brand. Only animal products have cholesterol.
- Even taking the fat off meats does not eliminate cholesterol. Cholesterol is found in the lean parts of meats as well as the fat.
- Shellfish and organ meats such as liver, kidney, and brains, and egg yolks are particularly high in cholesterol.

Most Americans are now eating between 600 and 800 milligrams of cholesterol every day. Many experts think that should be cut to at least 300 milligrams per day. Pritikin says on his extremely low fat diet, you only eat 100 milligrams of cholesterol per day.

By cutting down on animal and dairy fats, and eating more grains and vegetables—which do not have a smidgen of cholesterol and very little fat—you automatically reduce your intake of cholesterol radically.

Here is a list of the cholesterol content of some common foods:

Food	Amount	Cholesterol (Milligrams)
Milk, skim, fluid or reconstituted dry	1 cup	5
Cottage cheese, uncreamed	½ cup	7
Mayonnaise, commercial	1 tbsp	10
Lard	1 tbsp	12
Yogurt, made from fluid and dry nonfat milk, plain or vanilla	carton (227 gm)	17
Cream, light table	1 fl. oz.	20
Cottage cheese, creamed	½ cup	24
Cheese, pasteurized, processed American	28 gm (about 1 oz.)	25
Cheese, pasteurized, processed Swiss	28 gm (about 1 oz.)	26
Cream, half and half	¼ cup	26
Ice cream, regular, approximately 10% fat	½ cup	27
Cheese, cheddar	1 oz.	28
Milk, whole	1 cup	34
Sausage, frankfurter, all meat, cooked	1 frank	34
Butter	1 tbsp	35
Beef and vegetable stew, canned	1 cup	36
Cake, baked from mix, yellow 2 layer, made with eggs, water, chocolate frosting	75 gm	36
Oysters, salmon	3 oz., cooked	40
Clams, halibut, tuna	3 oz., cooked	55
Chicken, turkey, light meat	3 oz., cooked	67
Beef, pork, lobster, chicken, turkey, dark meat	3 oz., cooked	75
Lamb, veal, crab	3 oz., cooked	85
Tuna, canned in oil, drained solids	184 gm	116
Lobster, cooked, meat only	145 gm	123
Shrimp	3 oz., cooked	130
Heart, beef	3 oz., cooked	230
Egg	1 yolk or 1 egg	250

Food	Amount	Cholesterol (Milligrams)
Liver, beef, calf, hog, lamb	3 oz., cooked	370
Kidney	3 oz., cooked	680
Brains	3 oz., raw	more than 1700

Source: U.S. Department of Agriculture

CAN YOU EAT TOO LITTLE FAT?

Perhaps it is possible to eat dangerously low amounts of fat if you're on a near-starvation diet, but the possibility is very remote for ordinary American eaters. Studies have shown that both adults and youngsters on a highly controlled synthetic diet of only 1 percent (in linoleic acid) showed no ill effects during a six-month to two-year trial. The fact is virtually no foods are totally absent of fat, so you are bound to get some fat if you eat at all. For example, blackberries have one fat gram per cup, as do dried beans. Nearly all fruits, vegetables and grains have at least traces of fat, even lettuce. So it is impossible to eat a no-fat diet of ordinary foods and stay alive.

One question sometimes raised is: Will I get enough protein if I cut down on fatty foods? Protein deficiency has never been a problem in this country, except among the exceedingly undernourished. Most people get far more protein than they need, especially from high fat animal products. But the notion you cannot eat a diet low in fat and consume enough protein and other nutrients is a myth. Many low fat dairy products, such as dry cottage cheese, yogurt, skim milk have high amounts of protein. Taking away their fat grams does not destroy their protein value. One cup of skim milk provides 20 percent of the adult recommended daily allowances for protein and has practically no fat. One cup of evaporated skim milk offers 40 percent of your daily protein requirement. One-half cup of dry cottage cheese (with one gram of fat) provides 40 percent of your daily protein needs. Similarly, chicken and fish are high in protein and low in fat. Three ounces of crab meat has 35 percent of the daily protein needs and two grams of fat.*

* For a more comprehensive overview of the nutrients in various foods, see *Brand Name Nutrition Counter* by Jean Carper, Bantam Books.

Grains and vegetables contain small amounts of protein. The protein in these plant products is often termed "incomplete" because it lacks all the amino acids necessary to the body. However, as Frances Moore Lappé points out in her excellent book, *Diet for a Small Planet,* by combining certain foods, such as beans and rice, you can get a complete protein. She also notes that plant protein can be of quite high quality. She says when it comes to "net protein utilization" (the efficiency with which the body can use protein) rice and grains rank relatively high. For example, whole rice is on a par with meat in "net protein utilization." Experts generally say that if you're eating enough calories, you're probably getting enough protein.

What about other nutrients, such as vitamin A, which is fat-soluble? It is true that the fat in milk and butter carries high amounts of vitamin A, and that skim milk does not have significant amounts of vitamin A. However, that's not a problem if you eat a variety of other low fat foods. One cup of carrots has two to three times the recommended daily allowance of vitamin A, as does one cup of pumpkin, spinach or sweet potatoes. Grains do not ordinarily contain high levels of vitamin A, but most processed cereals on the market do because they are vitamin fortified. A serving of most cereals contains from 25 to 100 percent of the required vitamin A per day, as well as similar levels of several other nutrients.

Certainly a diet low in fat, like other type diets, could be dangerously deficient in nutrients if you do not eat a *variety* of foods. But, if you do that, you are *more* likely to get the necessary nutrients on a low fat diet than on a high fat one, according to Senator McGovern's nutrition committee. The reason, as the committee concluded, is that fats are "relatively poor sources of micronutrients, particularly in view of the calories they induce." In other words, per calorie, fatty foods have fewer nutrients; that is, they have a lower nutrient density. When you're trying to keep your weight down, you especially need to maximize the nutrients per calorie. One way to do it is by eating low fat foods.

According to McGovern's committee, when you eat a high fat diet you often replace highly nutritious carbohydrates with less nutritious fatty calories. Thus, the committee said: "Increased consumption of fruit, vegetables and whole grains is important with respect to supplying adequate amounts of vitamins and minerals and micronutrients"—trace minerals, such as chromium and selenium which are vital to health.

One other pointer: It is better to eat *whole* grain breads and cereals and brown rice, simply because they provide more nutrients than highly processed white flour products and white rice. This is equally true whether you are on a low fat or high fat diet.

A diet low in fat can be a vegetarian diet, but it need not be. You can still eat meat, just less of it, and it should be lean, well-trimmed of fat. For example, heart and cancer specialist Dr. Wynder says he eats red meat only once a week. You can also eat chicken, turkey and fish, all of which are low in fat, as long as they are not drenched in sauces or fried.

One caution: Do not cut down on fat by totally restricting yourself to only a few foods or one food, such as rice. This could be dangerous because it deprives your body of essential nutrients. If you have any doubts, consult your physician. Also, being on a low fat diet does not mean you can never eat high fat foods. You can, as long as you balance them out with low fat foods. Remember, it is not one or two fatty foods that matter; it is the *total* amount of fat in your diet that counts.

Visual Meat Portions and their Fat Units—Exact Size
Source U.S. Department of Agriculture

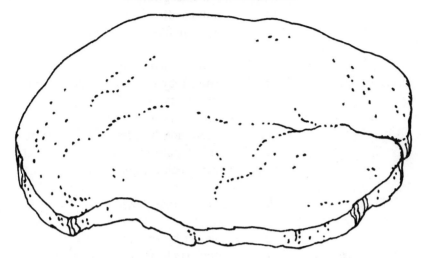

1. Roast Beef, lean. Two slices (single size shown above), 3 ounces cooked equals 4 fat units (each slice 4⅛ long, 2¼ wide, ¼ thick)

2. Chuck Roast, lean. One piece, 3 ounces cooked equals 2 fat units (one piece 2½ long, 2½ wide, ¾ thick)

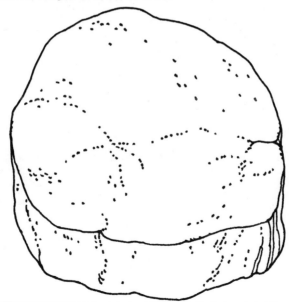

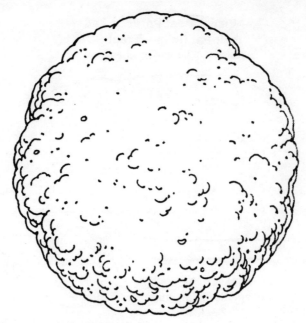

3. Hamburger, very lean beef. One hamburger, 3 ounces cooked equals 3½ fat units (diameter 3 inches, ⅝ thick)

4. Lamb Chops, lean. Two chops (single size shown above), 3 ounces cooked equals 2 fat units (each chop 4⅛ long, 2¼ wide, ¼ thick)

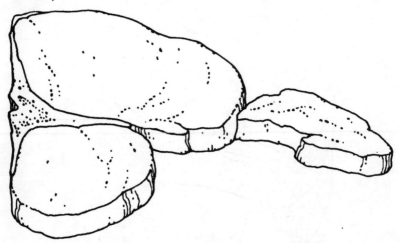

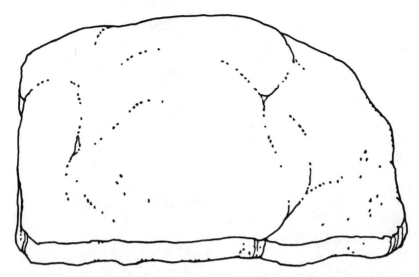

5. Ham, all fat removed. Two slices (single size shown above), 3 ounces cooked equals 3 fat units (each slice 4⅛ long, 2¼ wide, ¼ thick)

6. Roast Pork, all fat removed. One piece, 3 ounces cooked equals 4½ fat units (one piece 2½ long, 2½ wide, ¾ thick)

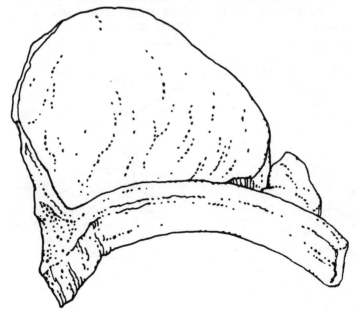

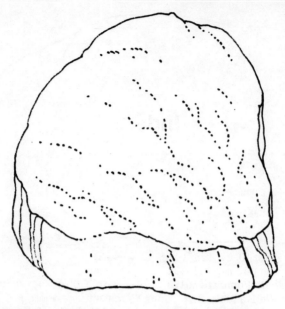

7. Veal Cutlet or Roast, lean. One piece, 3 ounces cooked equals 4½ fat units (one piece 2½ long, 2½ wide, ¾ thick)

8. Roast Turkey or Roast Chicken, light meat. Two slices (single size shown above), 3 ounces equals 1½ fat units (each slice 4 long, 2 wide, ¼ thick)

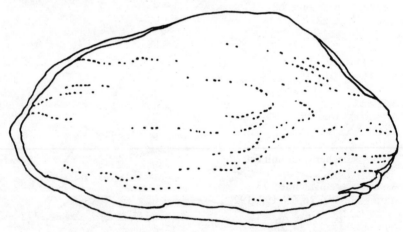

NOTE: USDA figures show a wide variance in the fat content in different cuts of beef.

Index